Qualitative Research for

IMMY HOLLOWAY
PhD, MA, BEd
Reader in Social Science

and

STEPHANIE WHEELER
BSc, RN, RM, RHV
Senior Lecturer in Nursing

INSTITUTE OF HEALTH AND COMMUNITY STUDIES
BOURNEMOUTH UNIVERSITY

b

Blackwell
Science

© 1996 by
Blackwell Science Ltd
Editorial Offices:
Osney Mead, Oxford OX2 0EL
25 John Street, London WC1N 2BL
23 Ainslie Place, Edinburgh EH3 6AJ
238 Main Street, Cambridge,
  Massachusetts 02142, USA
54 University Street, Carlton,
  Victoria 3053, Australia

Other Editorial Offices:
Arnette Blackwell SA
  224, Boulevard Saint Germain
  75007 Paris, France

Blackwell Wissenschafts-Verlag GmbH
  Kurfürstendamm 57
  10707 Berlin, Germany

  Zehetnergasse 6
  A-1140 Wien
  Austria

First published 1996

Set in 10/13 Ehrhardt
by DP Photosetting, Aylesbury, Bucks
Printed and bound in Great Britain by
Hartnolls Ltd, Bodmin, Cornwall

DISTRIBUTORS

Marston Book Services Ltd
PO Box 87
Oxford OX2 0DT
(*Orders:* Tel: 01865 791155
        Fax: 01865 791927
        Telex: 837515)

USA
Blackwell Science, Inc.
238 Main Street
Cambridge, MA 02142
(*Orders:* Tel: 800 215-1000
        617 876-7000
        Fax: 617 492-5263)

Canada
Copp Clark, Ltd
2775 Matheson Blvd East
Mississanga, Ontario
Canada, L4W 4P7
(*Orders:* Tel: 800 263-4374
        905 238-6074)

Australia
Blackwell Science Pty Ltd
54 University Street
Carlton, Victoria 3053
(*Orders:* Tel: 03 9347-0300
        Fax: 03 9349 3016)

A catalogue record for this book is available from the
British Library

ISBN 0–632–03765–2

Library of Congress
Cataloging-in-Publication Data
Holloway, Immy,
    Qualitative research for nurses/Immy Holloway
and Stephanie Wheeler.
       p.   cm.
    Includes bibliographical references and index.
    ISBN 0-632-03765-2
1. Nursing—Research—Methodology.
I. Wheeler, Stephanie. II. Title.
    [DNLM: 1. Nursing Research—methods.
    WY 20.5 H745q 1996]
RT81.5.H656   1996
610.73'072—dc20
DNLM/DLC
for Library of Congress   95-26498
                                              CIP

Contents

Foreword

Qualitative methods are appropriate for the study of many areas of nursing practice, education and policy. There is no such thing as a best method, it is of course a matter of fit between the issue in question and the method which will help to shed light upon it.

Qualitative methods have over the last decade or so moved from their home in sociology and anthropology out into health care and other more practice orientated areas. This is to be welcomed, it does however bring with it problems. Subtle questions of epistemology which were well understood in their original home disciplines are often lost in the unhelpful uncoupling of the practicalities of research methods from their philosophical and epistemological underpinnings which often occurs in the writing of introductory methods texts. Not so here!

This is a timely book and a fine addition to the literature on qualitative methods because it offers a lucid approach which will allow newcomers to the field to avoid the dislocation of methods from their theoretical bases. Those contemplating research of a qualitative nature will find here a discussion of a range of methods which can be described as qualitative. They will also find a good deal of discussion and debate, particularly useful are the sections on phenomenology and triangulation – areas where, in my view, most damage is done in the name of qualitative methodology.

Immy Holloway and Stephanie Wheeler have brought their considerable combined talents to this work and the result is a very readable introduction to what is a complex area. The inclusion of rather more of a philosophical discussion than one might expect to find in such a text is appropriate as it is the omission of just such discussion which leads to over simplification of methods which is ultimately unhelpful.

Undergraduates in a variety of health related fields should find this not only a good introduction to qualitative methods but also a very useful reference work for future use. The book is well presented and draws upon a wide range of work. The bibliography is itself an extremely valuable part of the book.

I imagine that this will become a 'must have' on the reading lists of those of us charged with teaching qualitative methods. Holloway and Wheeler have not shied away from some of the more contentious debates in qualitative methods and by taking the approach that they have, I suspect that they will find a readership among some of the older hands as well as those coming new to the area.

I can do no more than to encourage you to read on, further exhortation on my part serves only to hold you back from this tour de force.

Professor Kath M. Melia
B Nurs (Manc), PhD
Chair of Nursing Studies, University of Edinburgh

Preface

Overview

This book is intended for three main groups:

(1) Undergraduates, especially mature students who have nursing and midwifery experience
(2) Pre-registration nursing and midwifery students with some appreciation of research methods
(3) Post-graduates who undertake a qualitative research project and wish to revisit the procedures and strategies of qualitative research

The aim of this book is to provide nurses and midwives with theoretical understanding and practical knowledge of the qualitative research process. To achieve this, we have not only explained practical procedures but also the theoretical concepts which underlie qualitative research. We realise that novice researchers might find some of the issues rather complex.

In our experience researchers often undertake projects in a vacuum without considering the theoretical basis of their research and the origins of the approach they use. We have tried therefore to provide the theoretical background to some of these approaches. This accounts for the variation in length and complexity in the different chapters of the book.

We hope that the chapters will help researchers in nursing and midwifery to understand the different approaches, to present a proposal and to write the research report.

Chapter 1 describes the nature of qualitative enquiry and explains its position in the wider framework of research. In the following chapters we outline the steps in the research process from its initial stages of formulating the research question to writing a proposal. Access and entry to the setting and participants are discussed (Chapters 2 and 3). Chapter 3 deals with the ethical requirements that must be fulfilled and the philosophical framework on which they are based.

The next section gives an overview and practical guidelines for data collection (Chapters 4 and 5). We also discuss the major research approaches in greater detail and briefly outline others (Chapters 6–11). The issues of trustworthiness and authenticity in this type of enquiry are debated in Chapter 12. Chapter 13 gives guidelines for writing up the research.

The final section of the book deals with problems and supervision issues

(Chapters 14 and 16). As some qualitative researchers analyse their data by computer we include a chapter with a brief outline on their use (Chapter 15).

How to use the book

Students need not read the whole book from start to finish, although this would help them to understand the nature of qualitative research. It is essential, however, for those who are undertaking a research project to study Chapters 1, 2, 3, 4, 12 and 13. In addition they should read the chapter on their chosen approach. References at the end of this chapter will provide guidance for further reading.

We have tried in the references to include both classic texts and up-to-date books and articles on each area of qualitative research. This, and the wish to give all the sources used by us, is the reason for the extensive referencing.

Doing research is a challenging and demanding activity. We hope you will also enjoy it.

The authors

Although this book is the work of both of us, we complement each other in our knowledge and skills. Immy Holloway has a special interest in grounded theory and ethnography, and in the practicalities of doing and writing up research. Stephanie Wheeler, with a nursing, midwifery and health visiting background, is a specialist in health care ethics and law and has an interest in philosophy and the debate about 'validity' in qualitative research.

Dr Immy Holloway is a Reader in the Institute of Health and Community Studies at Bournemouth University and a sociologist of health and illness.

Stephanie Wheeler is Senior Lecturer in Nursing and theme leader for health care ethics and law in the same department.

Acknowledgements

We would like to thank Lisa Field, our editor, for her help, encouragement and patience throughout the writing of this book.

We are also indebted to a number of other people:

Dr Janet Walker, Health Psychologist, Reader in Health Studies, King Alfred's College, Winchester, our colleague and friend, whose constructive comments on the early drafts helped us a great deal.

Janice Clarke, Lecturer in the Department of Nursing at the University of Southampton, for her support.

Steven P. Wainwright, Lecturer at King's College, London University, for his detailed and constructive critique of most chapters of the book.

And last, but not least, our colleagues who gave us moral support throughout.

Immy Holloway and *Stephanie Wheeler*

Chapter 1

The Nature of Qualitative Research

In this chapter we aim to discuss:

- The historical background
- The reasons for qualitative research in nursing
- The main features of qualitative research
- The qualitative–quantitative debate

Two major approaches to research exist, qualitative and quantitative enquiry. These can be complementary or conflicting. Qualitative research is based on the belief that knowledge is socially constructed. Those who use this framework acknowledge that both researchers and the people they research have their own values and realities, therefore multiple realities exist.

Qualitative methods focus on the everyday life of people, although a variety of labels exist for this type of research (Hammersley & Atkinson, 1995). Other terms include fieldwork, interpretive research, naturalistic enquiry or case study approaches. Although there are differences between qualitative research methods (Baker *et al.*, 1992; Stern, 1994) it would be difficult to find clear distinctions between all of these approaches.

As a form of enquiry, qualitative research can be used in any social science or health care discipline. It has frequently been used in nursing and social work, as well as in sociology, anthropology and psychology.

Historical background

There has been increased interest in qualitative approaches to research among nurses and midwives since the 1970s. These approaches are not new; indeed, they were initially based on the methods used in anthropology and the *Chicago School* of sociology, and their roots lie in a journalistic and social work approach (Fielding, 1993), although journalistic methods have long been abandoned by qualitative researchers because they were seen as lacking in rigour.

Sociologists and anthropologists maintain that the qualitative researchers study people in their natural settings (Lincoln & Guba, 1985; Fielding, 1993). They look at individuals and groups in their settings, in order to discover the social world of cultures and languages by living with the 'natives' and learn by observing and talking to them. The Chicago School of the 1920s and 1930s (a group of sociologists of whom the most famous was Robert Park) transferred anthropological methods to western culture and society. The Chicagoans reported from 'the field' – the street corners, slums and drinking places of the city – feeling impelled to take part in the life of the informants to understand their reality. Data were collected from *participant observation* (a term coined by Lindemann, 1924, which means that the researcher participated in the culture under study) and informal interviews that produced lively and interesting stories from those who were observed.

For the research to be real, the Chicago sociologists recognised that they had to collect empirical data, 'to get their hands dirty'. Today's sociologists and psychologists too, know that the collection of data from different times and places assists in increasing understanding of our own society and social behaviour.

Qualitative research is especially useful where little is known about the area of study and the particular problem, setting or situation, because the research can reveal processes that go beyond surface appearances. It provides fresh and new perspectives on known areas and ideas (Strauss & Corbin, 1990). Some of the major approaches and their origins are given in Fig. 1.1.

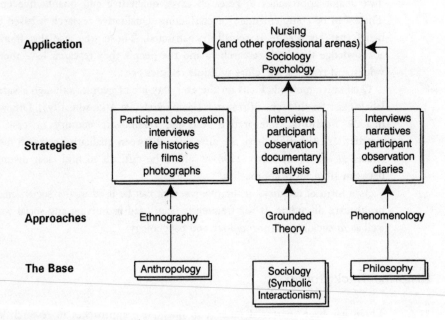

Fig. 1.1 Three major interpretative approaches.

The reasons for doing qualitative nursing research

Qualitative researchers adopt a person–centred and holistic perspective. The approach develops understanding of human experiences which is important for health professionals who focus on caring, communication and interaction. Through this approach, nurse and midwife researchers gain rich knowledge and insight about human beings – be they patients, colleagues or other professionals. Researchers generate an in-depth account which presents a lively picture of the participants' reality. The method focuses on human beings within their social and cultural context, not just on specific conditions. It is in tune with the nature of the phenomena examined: emotions, perceptions and actions are qualitative experiences.

Nurses and midwives have long recognised that individuals are more than body systems or diagnostic cases (Leininger, 1985), and therefore research must focus on the whole person rather than merely on a physical part. The nurse, taking a holistic view, looks at people in their natural environment, and the researcher–informant relationship is based on trust and openness. Both nursing and qualitative research depend on knowledge of the social context. The setting in which individuals live or stay for a time, the social support they have, and the people with whom they interact, have a powerful effect on their lives.

One could claim that a 'fit' exists between nursing philosophy and qualitative research. The essence of modern nursing contains elements of commitment and patience, understanding and trust, give and take, flexibility and openness (Paterson, 1978). These traits mirror those of qualitative enquiry with an emphasis on process, closeness to the data and openmindedness. Indeed, Morse (1994) focuses on the fact that flexibility is crucial to qualitative study. In the clinical setting as in qualitative research, the nurse has to 'backtrack', return to the situation and 'try something new' because the situation constantly evolves.

The main features of qualitative research

Different types of qualitative research approaches have some characteristics and procedures in common, while certain differences in data collection and analysis exist.

The following elements are common to most qualitative methods

(1) Qualitative research takes the 'emic' perspective, the insider's point of view
(2) Researchers immerse and involve themselves in the setting and the culture under study
(3) The data have primacy; the theoretical framework is not predetermined by the data but derives from it
(4) The method includes 'thick description'
(5) The relationship between the researcher and the researched is close and is based on a position of equality as human beings.
(6) Data collection and analysis interact

We will now discuss these in greater detail.

The 'emic' perspective

Qualitative researchers explore the ideas and perceptions of the participants, the insider's view. This is called the 'emic' perspective by anthropologists and linguists (Harris, 1976). It means that researchers attempt to examine the experiences, feelings and perceptions of the people they study rather than imposing a framework of their own which might distort the ideas of the participants. They uncover the meanings people give to their experiences and the way in which they interpret them. Qualitative research is based on the premise that individuals are best placed to describe situations and feelings in their own words. It must be stressed though that these meanings are seldom clear or unambiguous (Addison, 1992), and they are not fixed; the social world is not frozen at a particular point in time or in a particular situation but dynamic and changing.

By observing people and listening to their accounts, researchers seek to understand the process by which participants make sense of their own behaviour and the rules which govern their practices. This means taking into account their intentions because they help researchers gain access to their social reality. Of course, the reports individuals give are *their* explanations, which may not always be *the* explanation of an event or action, but as the researcher wishes to uncover the individual's own definition of reality, these reports are valid data. Although Dey (1993) warns us that we cannot always rely on accounts or on our own interpretations of them, we can often take our informants' words and actions as reflections of underlying meanings.

The qualitative approach requires *empathetic understanding*, that is, the investigators must try to examine the situations, events and actions from the participants' (the social actors') point of view and not impose their own perspective. This does not mean that the researchers never theorise or infer from observed behaviour or participants' words – they often do. The researchers' and outsiders' view is the 'etic' perspective (Harris, 1976). They interpret the ideas of the participants and give an account of events and actions. There is 'elaboration and systematisation of the significance of an identified phenomenon' (Banister *et al.*, 1994:3). Meanings are not reduced to purely subjective accounts. The participants are part of the group or subculture in which they live, and therefore their words, actions and intentions can only be understood in context. The health professionals who research them have access to their world through experience and observation and interpret their words and actions.

It is necessary that the relationship between researcher and informant is one of trust; this close relationship and the researcher's in-depth knowledge of the informants' situation makes deceit unlikely (though not impossible).

Immersion in the setting

Most qualitative research investigates patterns of interaction or seeks knowledge about a group or a culture. In the clinical setting this may be interaction between health professionals and clients or relatives, or interaction with colleagues. The culture or subculture may be a ward environment, the operating theatre, the reception area or indeed the community. It does not just consist of the physical environment but also of particular ideologies, values and ways of thinking that permeate the setting. Researchers need sensitivity to interpret what they observe and hear. Human beings are influenced by their experiences; therefore qualitative methods encompass processes and changes over time.

Immersion might mean attending meetings with or about participants, becoming familiar with other, similar situations, reading documents or observing interaction in the setting even before starting the research.

Example

Two nurses decide to explore patients' and nurses' feelings about mixed wards. They cannot just interview individuals out of context, but must visit mixed wards in different localities, read about them and listen to clients' and professionals' descriptions of them as well as observe interactions that go on in the setting.

For the understanding of participants' interpretations, it is necessary to become familiar with their world. When nurses or midwives do research, they are already part of the setting and know it intimately. This might mean, however, that they are over-familiar and could miss important issues or considerations. To be able to examine the world of the participant, the health professional must not take this world for granted, but must question his or her own assumptions and act like a stranger to the setting.

Example

A midwife tutor felt that the rule 'nil by mouth' shortly before the birth of a baby was distressing for clients who sometimes went for long periods without food or drink. All her colleagues had seen this as an important issue in the setting. She wished to develop a small research project on this topic and asked clients about their feelings concerning this rule. Even in her first few interviews and observations she found that clients had no opinion or concern about this, they were far more worried about their babies and the birth process. She had to abandon her research project.

It is important to remember that researchers have to take into account the total context of the data. The conditions in which they are gathered, the locality, the time and history are all important. Qualitative research is often called naturalistic enquiry (Lincoln & Guba, 1985; Erlandson *et al.*, 1993) for these very reasons. It means that events and actions are studied as they occur in everyday real life settings, and researchers must respect the context and culture in which they are involved and not try to change it while examining it. If researchers understand the context, they can locate the actions and perceptions of individuals and grasp the meanings which they communicate to us. The researcher as an active participant in the research process is the main research tool.

The primacy of data

Nurses and midwives in the clinical setting usually approach people with a view to finding out about them in order to assess them and plan care. The research process works in a similar way: researchers go to the participants to collect the rich and deep data which may become the basis for theorising. The data themselves generate ideas or help modify already existing theories. It means that the design cannot be strictly pre-defined. Qualitative research data have priority, whereas in other types of research, hypotheses are formed, sampling frames are imposed and theories set up to be tested. Although qualitative approaches are rooted in a specific theoretical background, for instance, philosophy or symbolic interactionism, the theoretical framework of the research project is not predetermined but based on the emerging data. Researchers do not impose assumptions but give analytic accounts of reality. This means that they must be open minded although they cannot help having some ideas about the research. Fetterman (1989:11) claims that the researcher 'enters the field with an open mind, not an empty head'.

The data are the words and actions of the participants gained through conversations and observations as well as documents and diaries.

Example

A nurse wanted to explore the perceptions and feelings of patients with multiple sclerosis. She interviewed them and asked them to keep diaries about the development or remission of their condition. These diaries and interviews become part of the data and could form the baseline for qualitative analysis.

While the aim of much qualitative research is the generation of theory (Glaser & Strauss, 1967), many researchers do not achieve this, particularly if they are novices. New ideas can emerge from the data; propositions or typologies are developed, but the researchers cannot state that they have generated theory unless this claim is substantiated. They usually do provide, however, the interpretation of participants' experiences and gain insights into their world, describing 'the characteristics and structure of the phenomenon' (Tesch 1991:22) they examined. Qualitative research is not static but developmental and dynamic in character.

Thick description

Immersion in the setting will help the researcher use *thick description* (Geertz, 1973). It involves detailed portrayals of the participants' experiences, going beyond a report of surface phenomena to their interpretations, uncovering feelings in a situation and the meanings of their actions. Thick description develops from the data and the context. The task involves description of the location and the people within it, giving visual pictures of setting, events and situations as well as verbatim narratives of individuals' accounts of their perceptions and ideas in context.

Example

In a small observational study. Ward (1990) described the reception of patients in an accident and emergency department. He gives a clear visual picture of the ways in which patients fill their waiting time, and how nurses or doctors call patients to the treatment area. The study shows patterns of interaction in the context of a reception area. Two excerpts show the liveliness and detail of this type of description: 'On a couple of occasions, just a head appeared around the door to call a name' and, 'when staff came out into the waiting room to call in patients, they tended to come as far as an invisible line drawn from the edge of the reception desk'.

The description of the situation or discussion should be thorough; this means that everything is described in vivid detail. Indeed Denzin (1989b:83) defines thick description as:

> 'deep, dense, detailed accounts of problematic experiences ... It presents detail, context, emotion and the webs of social relationship that join persons to one another.'

Thick description contains theoretical ideas about the importance of conduct and events, it is not merely factual but theoretical and analytic description. Strauss & Corbin (1994) go further by explaining that the emphasis in one of the approaches, grounded theory, is on conceptualisation rather than description.

Denzin (1989a) contrasts thick description with thin description, which is superficial and lacks detail (see Chapter 6). Thick description helps the reader of a research study to develop an active role in the research because knowledge is shared by researcher and reader. Through clear description of the culture or subculture, the context and the process of the research, the reader can follow the pathway of the researcher and the two share the construction of reality coming to similar conclusions in the analysis of research (Erlandson *et al.*, 1993). This shows readers of the story what they themselves would experience if they were in the same situation as the participants, and therefore thick description generates empathetic and experiential understanding.

Qualitative approaches are connected with observing, questioning and listening. This generates description of a culture by the researchers who immerse themselves in the real world of the participants (Hammersley & Atkinson, 1995). It helps to focus on process, on the interaction of people and the way they construct or change rules and situations. Qualitative enquiry can trace progress and development over time as perceived by the participants.

The research relationship

This is also discussed in Chapters 3 and 9.

Some essential characteristics of the health professional help to establish a relationship with the participants; indeed, these are the same qualities which nurses and midwives need in the caring relationship with their patients and clients. Rose (1994) claims that the research interview has similarities to nursing assessments: nurses gain information by talking to patients, listening and interpreting what they hear. Another similarity exists: nurses and patients generally share common overall aims, and in qualitative research this is also true for the researchers and participants (Schutz, 1994).

The following characteristics are important, and researchers should be:

• Good listeners
• Non-judgmental
• Friendly
• Open and honest
• Flexible

The reflective practitioner becomes a reflective listener. This involves a non-judgmental stance towards the thoughts and words of the participants. Swanson (1986) advises that researchers should reassure the participants that there is no right or wrong answer, which is particularly important when interviewing patients. Rapport and empathy help in uncovering rich data. In fact, the listener becomes the learner in this situation, while the informant is the teacher. Field & Morse (1985) remind us to show genuine interest in order to develop trust. This means keeping eye contact and being friendly without forgetting the purpose of the research. Rapport does not automatically imply an intimate relationship or deep friendship (Spradley, 1979), but it does lead to negotiation and sharing of ideas. It makes the research more interesting for the participants because they feel able to ask questions.

Questions about the nature of the research project should be answered as honestly and openly as possible without creating bias in the study. The advice is to tell the truth without going into detail which informants might not understand or which may frighten them (Bogdewic, 1992). It is interesting that research books and articles differ in their advice on the relationship of researcher and informant. Some (for instance Patton, 1990) suggest a certain distance between the two, while others, such as Wilde (1992) feel that this could be a mistake because involvement and self-disclosure on the part of the researcher facilitates disclosure and sharing of experiences from the participants. For nurses and midwives, we feel it is important that participants realise that researchers, too, have human experiences and can empathise with them. It is still important to remember the main goal of the meeting between researcher and informants – that is to gain knowledge which will improve clinical practice.

The interaction of data collection and analysis

Another important feature of qualitative research is the close connection between data collection and analysis. Without setting up a hypothesis prior to the study, the researchers collect the first data in the field and start to analyse them at the same time. They then develop tentative working propositions which are reformulated and modified in subsequent data collection. New concepts are developed throughout the process of data collection until the end of the research, and they are continuously adapted. When asking questions of new informants or looking at new situations, researchers take into account the ideas that emerged previously. New data may challenge or modify these. At each stage data collection and analysis interact.

The qualitative–quantitative debate: underlying philosophies

Social reality can be approached in different ways. Nurses and midwives will have to choose between a variety of research methods. While they often make their choice on practical grounds, they must also understand the philosophical ideas on which it is based. The approach depends on the following:

- The nature and type of research problem
- The epistemological stance of the researcher
- The skills and training of the researcher
- The resources available for the research project

Students, of course, have to think of the practicalities of the research, such as their own skills and interest, the scope of the research and available funds and resources; these are all factors which may influence the undertaking of a project. Qualitative research studies can be small-scale and cheap, whereas large surveys are expensive.

The initial choice of method is not easy. Approaches to social enquiry consist not only of the procedures of sampling, data collection and analysis, but they are based on particular ideas about the world and the nature of knowledge which sometimes reflect conflicting and competing views about social reality. Some of these interpretations of the social world are concerned with the very nature of existence (ontology). From this, basic assumptions about knowledge arise. Epistemology is the theory of knowledge. Minichiello *et al.* (1990:102) state: 'Epistemological issues are concerned with knowing or deciding what sort of statements we will accept to justify what we believe to exist'. Methodology refers to the principles and ideas on which researchers base their procedures and strategies.

In the following section we will discuss the epistemology of research approaches.

Epistemological concerns

Two main sets of assumptions underlie social research: the positivist and the interpretivist paradigms (Lincoln & Guba, 1985; Bryman, 1988). Conflict and

Table 1.1   Qualitative and quantitative research

	Qualitative	Quantitative
Aim	Exploration of participants' meaning Understanding, generation of theory from data	Search for causal explanations Testing hypothesis, prediction, control
Approach	Broad focus Process-orientated Context-bound, mostly natural setting Getting close to the data	Narrow focus Product-orientated Context-free, often in artificial setting
Sample	Participants, informants Sampling units such as place, time and concepts Flexible sampling which develops during research	Respondents, subjects Sample frame fixed before research starts
Data collection	In-depth non-standardised interviews Participant observation/fieldwork Documents, photographs, videos	Questionnaire, standardised interviews Tightly structured observation Documents Randomised controlled trials
Analysis	Thematic, latent content analysis Grounded theory, ethnographic analysis, etc.	Statistical analysis
Outcome	A story, an ethnography, a theory	Measurable results
Relationships	Direct involvement of researcher Research relationship close	Limited involvement of researcher Research relationship distant
Validity	Trustworthiness, authenticity	Internal/external validity, reliability

tension between different schools of social science have existed for a long time. In the positivist approach, the focus was on the methods of natural science which became a model for early social sciences such as psychology and later sociology. Interpretivists stressed that human beings differ from the material world and the distinction between humans and matter should be mirrored in the methods of investigation.

Positivism: the natural science model

In the past, the traditional and favoured method of social and behavioural research used was quantitative. Quantitative research is based on the positivist and early natural science paradigm which has influenced social science throughout the nineteenth and the first half of the twentieth centuries. Experimental research and survey research have their roots in this approach.

Positivism is an approach to science based on a belief in universal laws and insistence on objectivity and neutrality (Thompson, 1995). Positivists follow the natural science approach in which theories and hypotheses are tested. The methods of natural, in particular physical, science stem from the eighteenth and nineteenth centuries. Comte (1798–1857), the French philosopher, suggested that the emerging social sciences must proceed in the same way as natural science by adopting the natural science method of observation and experimentation as opposed to speculation or theological explanations of phenomena.

One of the rules in this type of research is the quest for objectivity and distance so that personal biases can be avoided. Investigators searched for patterns and regularities and believed that universal laws and rules or law-like generalities exist for human action. They thought that generalisations would be applicable to all situations or cases (Hitchcock & Hughes, 1989) making certain assumptions about human beings. Behaviour could be predicted, so they believed, on the basis of these laws. Even today many researchers think that numerical measurement, statistical analysis and the search for cause and effect lie at the heart of all research. They feel that detachment and objectivity are possible, and numerical measurement results in objective knowledge. In this approach, the researchers control the theoretical framework, sampling frames and the structure of the research.

Duffy (1985), declares that this type of research seeks causal relationships or links between events. Popper (1959) claimed that falsifiability is the main criterion of science. The researcher formulates a hypothesis, an expected outcome, and tests it. Experiments are designed or surveys set up to refute or falsify this hypothesis. Findings from observation or standardised interviews help to confirm or reject the hypothesis, but any statement must always be falsifiable. If it is disproved, the whole process starts anew. Particular cases have to *fit* the hypothesis. If *fit* exists and the hypothesis is not falsified the study is finished until the moment a deviant case occurs. The problem is that knowledge is always provisional. The main aim of this research is to test theory. This means that the approach develops from theory and the concepts are established before the research begins. The model of science adopted is hypothetico–deductive. The danger of this approach is that researchers treat perceptions of the social world as objective and absolute and neglect everyday subjective interpretations and the context of the research.

Social scientists must be reminded, however, that natural scientists, for instance biologists and physicists, are not agreed exactly on what science is and adopt a variety of different scientific methods. The popular, and traditional, idea of natural science is questioned by Chalmers (1982). The traditionalists believed that scientific knowledge can be proven, is discovered by rigorous methods of observation and experiments, and derived through the senses. Chalmers asserts that this is a simplistic view of science. Scientific knowledge is difficult to prove and is not merely derived from the senses. The search for objectivity may be futile for scientists; they may strive for it but their own biases, experiences and opinions intrude. Science, whether natural or social science, cannot be 'value free'.

In the 1960s the traditional view of science was attacked and criticised for its aims and methods, and its emphasis on social reality as being 'out there' separate from the individual. At this time, a *paradigm shift* (Kuhn, 1970) appears to have occurred. Natural scientists criticised the mechanical natural science view of the world and some sociologists began to see it as socially constructed and defined. The latter resurrected the interpretive perspective which initially stemmed from the writings of Mead and others in the early twentieth century. This is related to some of the ideas of the sociologist Weber (1864–1920).

The interpretive paradigm

The interpretive model has its roots in philosophy and the human sciences, particularly in history and anthropology. The approach centres on interpretation and the creation of meaning by human beings, and their subjective reality. They should be approached by scientists within the whole of their life context, not as individual entities who exist in a vacuum. Leininger (1985) stressed that knowledge of people consists of more than 'what can be seen, sensed and measured'. Social scientists who focus on this model believe that understanding human experiences is as important as the ideas of the positivist paradigm which focuses on explanation, prediction and control. This interpretive model has a long history (from nineteenth century historians to Weberian sociology) but it has gained more acceptance in the last few decades.

The interpretivist paradigm can be linked to Weber's *Verstehen* approach. Philosophers such as Dilthey (1833–1911) considered that the social sciences should not ape the natural sciences. Truzzi (1974:9) writes:

'Humanistic and artistic insights are the goals of the social sciences, and these are achieved not through the methods of the natural sciences but only by means of empathetic identification with the values and meanings examined in the minds of social actors'.

Weber too, was well aware of the two paradigms which existed in the 19th century. The concept of *Verstehen* (understanding something in its context) has elements of empathy, not in the psychological sense as intuitive and non-conscious feeling, but as reflexive reconstruction and interpretation of the action of others. Weber believed that social scientists should be concerned with the interpretive understanding of human beings. He claimed that meaning can be found in the intentions and goals of the individual.

Weber argued that *understanding* in the social sciences is inherently different from *explanation* in the natural sciences, and he differentiates between the nomothetic, rule-governed methods of the latter and the idiographic methods which are not linked to the general laws of nature but to the actions of human beings. Weber believed that numerically measured probability is quantitative only, and he wanted to stress that social science concerns itself with the qualitative. We should treat the people we study, he advised, 'as if they were human beings' and try to gain access to their experiences and perceptions by listening to them and observing them.

Contemporary interpretivists claim that the experiences of people are essentially context-bound, that is they cannot be free from time and location or the mind of the human actor. Researchers must understand the socially constructed nature of the world and realise that values and interests become part of the research process. Objectivity and neutrality are impossible to achieve; in fact, the values of researchers and participants can become an integral part of the research (Smith,

1983). Researchers are not divorced from the phenomenon under study. This means reflexivity on their part; they must take into account their own position in the setting as they are the main research tool (see also Chapter 14).

Language itself is context-bound and depends on the researchers' and informants' values and social location. Replication or duplication of a piece of research is impossible because the research relationship, history and location of participants differ in each study. It is sometimes suggested that qualitative research is not scientific, though most qualitative researchers claim that it is (Hitchcock & Hughes, 1989; Minichiello *et al.*, 1990). Traditional nineteenth century methods of physical science are not the only way to do science. (This is discussed further in Chapter 14.)

Qualitative methodology is not completely precise nor does it generally use statistics and numerical values. Investigators in qualitative enquiry do begin with empirical data but turn to the human participants for guidance, control and direction throughout the research. Rigour and order are, of course, important, particularly when working with qualitative analysis. The social world is not orderly or systematic, therefore it is all the more important that the researcher proceeds in a well structured and systematic way.

Conflicting or complementary perspectives?

Some social scientists believe that qualitative and quantitative approaches are merely different ways for research to be used pragmatically, dependent on the research question, while others explore the epistemological bases of the two methodologies, decide that they are incompatible and mutually exclusive (this is debated in Hammersley, 1992), and use one or the other depending on their own epistemological stance. Bryman (1988) and Silverman (1993) address this by stating that neither school is superior to the other, and that an emphasis on the polarities does not result in useful debates. They do, however, stress that the approach depends on the intentions and goals of the researcher.

Many sociologists and psychologists still work in the positivist tradition. In clinical research, however, the qualitative perspective has been increasingly used. Guba & Lincoln (1981) argue that a paradigm shift (in line with the ideas of Kuhn, 1970) occurred when earlier methods of natural science were questioned and new ways adopted: certain theoretical and philosophical presuppositions are replaced by another set of assumptions taking precedence over the model from the past. Some, like Atkinson (1995), do not believe that qualitative methodology represents a shift to a new paradigm. However, we suggest that it is a coherent way of researching human thought, perception and behaviour (not new but more systematic and scientific than earlier ethnography or journalistic narrative).

Corner (1991) warns the researcher not to be simplistic about the assumptions of social science and overemphasise the differences between the methods which are based on these different philosophies. Nevertheless, it must be remembered that positivist and interpretive methods of social science have their roots in competing and conflicting ideas. While positivism is based on the belief that reality has existence outside and independent of individuals, interpretivists claim that reality is socially constructed and not independent of the observer (Blaikie, 1993).

Triangulation

Triangulation is the use of several methods (or data sources, theories or researchers) in the study of one phenomenon. The concept has its origin in ancient Greek mathematics; in modern times it is employed in topographic surveying as a checking system. Denzin (1989a) differentiates between four main types of triangulation: triangulation of data, investigators, theories and methodologies. The triangulation of methodologies is most often used.

In data triangulation researchers gain their data from different groups, locations and times. For example: in a study of hospitalisation, male and female patients' perspectives could be explored. The surgical and medical wards might be the locations in which the research takes place. An admission in the middle of the night could be compared with one during the day.

Investigator triangulation means that more than one researcher is involved in the research. In student projects, dissertations or theses this does not often happen, but some well-known researchers have used investigator triangulation. For instance, Strauss researched work in psychiatric hospitals with a number of other researchers (Strauss et al., 1964).

Theory triangulation (the use of different theoretical perspectives in the study of one problem) is rarer.

Usually researchers use methodological triangulation in its two main forms:

- Within-method (intra-method) triangulation
- Between-method (across-method or inter-method) triangulation

Within-method triangulation adopts different strategies but stays within a single paradigm. For instance, participant observation and open-ended interviews are often used together in one qualitative study. A good example of this is Becker's research (Becker et al., 1961). He and his co-workers studied new doctors in the hospital setting through observation and asked them about their work through non-standardised qualitative interviews.

Researchers use between-method triangulation to confirm the findings generated through one particular method by another. An example would be if a nurse constructed a questionnaire about a problem, but would also employ unstructured interviews to confirm the validity of the former. It is sometimes believed that triangulation can improve validity and overcome the biases inherent in one perspective However, Sarantakos (1993:156) claims that 'there is no evidence to suggest that studies based on triangulation produce necessarily more valid results', and that the desirability of triangulation depends on the particular project. Clarke (1995) goes further, stating that only those who have an over-optimistic picture of research try to demonstrate that triangulation between different methodologies is appropriate. We suggest to nurses or midwives who wish to triangulate, that this should be done only by experienced researchers who have employed qualitative and quantitative methods separately and are familiar with both.

Data triangulation is different from mixing methods. In triangulation, the researchers approach the same problem in different ways or from different angles. When they mix methods, they look at different problems in the same research study using different approaches.

Mixing methods

Sometimes researchers employ two methodologies which have their roots in distinctively different views of the world, not for validating the results of one through the other, but for different reasons, for instance to gain a variety of information, to illuminate a particular problem from different angles, or to look at different aspects of a phenomenon. DePoy & Gitlin (1993) describe the three basic techniques for mixing methods: the *nested*, the *sequential* and the *parallel* strategies.

(1) Using the *nested* strategy, researchers choose a main framework and methodology to develop their research and then add a technique from another methodology. For instance, a nurse might employ participant observation and then conduct a survey on a particular issue which arose during the data collection or in the findings.

(2) *Sequential* strategies can also be used. They are the most common approaches to mixing methods. Nurses, for example, often use qualitative techniques, such as unstructured interviewing, as a first step in research to explore an issue. On the basis of these interviews they develop a hypothesis and construct a questionnaire for a large survey. Sometimes, on the other hand, a study starts with a quantitative approach which examines facts, and a qualitative strategy is added to explore feelings and perceptions which have not been explored before in depth.

(3) The *parallel* approach makes use of the qualitative and the quantitative at the same time while valuing both equally so that the topic can be illuminated from all sides.

The debate about triangulation

Social scientists are not in accord about the use of triangulation and the mixing of methods. Hammersley (1992) denies the existence of two methodological models and claims that distinctions are dangerous. Although fundamental differences may exist in these approaches, researchers should also consider the implications of the methods for practice and operational use, where a clear distinction is not always helpful. Miles & Huberman (1994) state that one of the differences lies in the description in words in qualitative research and numbers in quantitative research, but there are, of course, differences in sampling, analysis and outcomes. Qualitative and quantitative methods are often used together in one single study for practical purposes, and some social scientists claim that a research study can be strengthened and improved through using both methods (Salomon, 1991).

Those with purist views suggest that the two main research methodologies have no place in one piece of research. Indeed, Leininger (1992) – who recognises that research findings from different philosophical directions can complement each other – warns researchers against mixing the two methodologies because they differ in philosophy, traits and aims. She does suggest that researchers mix methods *within* a paradigm. Triangulation *across* methods, which Leininger describes as *multiangulation*, violates the integrity of both methodologies in her view. Clarke (1995) advises against using multiple methodologies for more practical reasons. He states that this produces a diffused picture because of the lack of consistency and adequacy in analysis.

The practical angle should be considered: in a small undergraduate project a single method approach is less time consuming and gives an opportunity for in-depth use of the method. Cresswell (1994) recommends that studies be based on a single paradigm, not only because of the limitations of time and size of the research, but also because each methodology has its roots in a particular world view. Qualitative methods are appropriate for researching some situations and problems, quantitative methods for others. Researchers must choose the method or methods which best suit the research question or topic. Depending on a particular project, triangulation between methods may be appropriate.

Nurse researchers rarely adopt the purist stance but are more pragmatic. They do not necessarily see a conflict or follow an extremist view, a standpoint which would be irrelevant in nursing research. Evaluators of qualitative or quantitative methods must remember to judge each piece of work on its own terms within the specific approach taken. This becomes particularly important advice for qualitative research, which is often evaluated by the use of criteria appropriate for quantitative methods. Hutchinson & Webb (1991:311) note that 'qualitative research is not a substitute for quantitative inquiry. The two modes of research are not in competition'. Each has to be consistent within itself and fit the research topic or problem. While quantitative researchers stress validity, ensuring that instruments are appropriate and measure what they are supposed to measure, qualitative research is seen to have greater explanatory power. This indeed is its main strength.

Summary

Qualitative research focuses on the 'lived experience' and the interpretations and meaning which people attach to it. The researcher is the main research tool. Observation and interviews show how participants affect the social world and what factors and conditions influence them. Researchers therefore have to become immersed in the setting and situation of the informants and describe them in lively detail.

There is no initial hypothesis (although, of course, researchers have a hunch); ideas and theories are developed directly from the data which have primacy. Data collection and analysis interact from the beginning of the research. Qualitative research is useful for health professionals because it adopts a holistic person-centred perspective. Leininger (1992:409) states that 'grasping the totality of institutions, human environments, and life contexts, beliefs and values is a tremendous strength of qualitative studies'. This is what qualitative nursing and midwifery research attempts to do.

References

Addison R.B. (1992) Grounded hermeneutic research. In: *Doing Qualitative Research* (eds B.F. Crabtree & W.L. Miller), pp. 110–124, Sage, Newbury Park, California.

Atkinson P. (1995) Some perils of paradigms. *Qualitative Health Research*, **5** (1), 117–124

Baker C., Wuest J. & Stern P.N. (1992) Method slurring: the phenomenology/grounded theory example. *Journal of Advanced Nursing*, **7**, 1355–1360.

Banister P., Bruman E., Parker I., Taylor M. & Tindall C. (1994) *Qualitative Methods in Psychology: A Research Guide*. Open University Press, Milton Keynes.

Becker H.S., Geer B., Hughes E. & Strauss A.L. (1961) *Boys in White*. University of Chicago Press, New Brunswick.

Blaikie N.W. (1993) *Approaches to Social Enquiry*. Blackwell Science, Oxford.

Bogdewic S.P. (1992) Participant observation. In: *Doing Qualitative Research. Research Methods in Primary Care*, Volume 3 (eds B.F. Crabtree & W.L. Miller), pp. 45–69, Sage, Newbury Park, California.

Bryman A. (1988) *Quantity and Quality in Social Research*. Unwin Hyman, London.

Chalmers A.F. (1982) *What is this Thing called Science?* Open University Press, Milton Keynes.

Clarke L. (1995) Nursing research: science, visions and telling stories. *Journal of Advanced Nursing*, **21**, 584–593.

Corner J. (1991) In search of more complete answers to questions: quantitative versus qualitative methods, is there a way forward? *Journal of Advanced Nursing*, **16**, 718–727.

Cresswell J.W. (1994) *Qualitative and Quantitative Methods*. Sage, Newbury Park, California.

Denzin N.K. (1989a) *The Research Act: A Theoretical Introduction to Sociological Methods*, 3rd edn. Prentice-Hall, Englewood Cliffs, New Jersey.

Denzin N.K. (1989b) *Interpretive Interactionism*. Sage, Newbury Park, California.

DePoy E. & Gitlin L.N. (1993) *Introduction to Research: Multiple Strategies for Health and Human Services*. Mosby, St Louis.

Dey I. (1993) *Qualitative Data Analysis: A User-Friendly Guide for Social Scientists*. Routledge, London.

Duffy M.E. (1985) Designing nursing research: the qualitative–quantitative debate. *Journal of Advanced Nursing*, **10**, 225–231.

Erlandson D.A., Harris E.L., Skipper B.L. & Allen S.D. (1993) *Doing Naturalistic Research*. Sage, Newbury Park, California.

Fetterman D.M. (1989) *Ethnography: Step by Step*. Sage, Newbury Park, California.

Field P.A. & Morse J.M. (1985) *Nursing Research: The Application of Qualitative Approaches*. Croom Helm, London.

Fielding N. (1993) Ethnography. In: *Researching Social Life* (ed. N. Gilbert), pp. 154–171, Sage, London.

Geertz C. (1973) *The Interpretation of Cultures*. Basic Books, New York.

Glaser B. G. & Strauss A.L. (1967) *The Discovery of Grounded Theory: Strategies for Qualitative Research*. Aldine De Gruyter, New York.

Guba E.G. & Lincoln Y. (1981) Epistemological and methodological bases of naturalistic inquiry. *Educational Communication and Technology Journal*, **82** (30), 233–252.

Hammersley M. (1992) *What's Wrong with Ethnography?* Routledge, London.

Hammersley M. & Atkinson P. (1995) *Ethnography: Principles in Practice*, 2nd edn. Tavistock, London.

Harris M. (1976) History and significance of the emic/etic distinction. *Annual Review of Anthropology*, **5**, 329–350.

Hitchcock G. & Hughes D. (1989) *Research and the Teacher; A Qualitative Introduction to School-Based Research*. Routledge, London.

Hutchinson S. & Webb R. (1991) Teaching qualitative research. Perennial problems and possible solutions. In: *Qualitative Nursing Research: A Contemporary Dialogue* (ed. J.M. Morse), revised edn, pp. 301–321, Sage, Newbury Park, California.

Kuhn T.S. (1970) *The Structure of Scientific Revolutions*, 2nd edn. University of Chicago Press, Chicago.

Leininger M. (1985) *Qualitative Research Methods in Nursing*. Grune and Stratton, New York.

Leininger M. (1992) Current issues, problems, and trends to advance qualitative paradigmatic research methods for the future. *Qualitative Health Research*, **2** (4), 392–415.

Lincoln Y.S. & Guba E.G. (1985) *Naturalistic Inquiry*. Sage, Beverley Hills, California.

Lindemann E.C. (1924) *Social Discovery*. Republic, New York.

Miles M.B. & Huberman A.M. (1994) *Qualitative Data Analysis*, 2nd edn. Sage, Thousand Oaks, California.

Minichiello V., Aroni R., Timewell E. & Alexander L. (1990) *In-Depth Interviewing; Researching People*. Longman Cheshire, Melbourne.

Morse J.M. (1994) Motivational signs and symptoms. *Qualitative Health Research*, **4** (3) 259–261.

Paterson J.A. (1978) cited in Munhall P.L. & Oiler C. (1986) *Nursing Research; A Qualitative Perspective*. Appleton Century Crofts, New York.

Patton M.Q. (1990) *Qualitative Evaluation and Research Methods*, 2nd edn. Sage, Newbury Park, California.

Popper K. (1959) *The Logic of Scientific Discovery*. Routledge & Keegan Paul, London.

Rose K. (1994) Unstructured and semi-structured interviewing. *Nurse Researcher*, **1** (3) 23–29.

Salomon G. (1991) Transcending the qualitative–quantitative debate: the analytic and systematic approaches to educational research. *Educational Research*, **20**, 10–18.

Sarantakos S. (1993) *Social Research*. Macmillan, Basingstoke.

Schutz S.E. (1994) Exploring the benefits of a subjective approach in qualitative nursing research. *Journal of Advanced Nursing* **20**, 412–417.

Silverman D. (1993) *Interpreting Qualitative Data*. Sage, London.

Smith J.K. (1983) Quantitative versus qualitative research: an attempt to clarify the issue. *Educational Researcher*, **12** (3), 6–13.

Spradley J.P. (1979) *The Ethnographic Interview*. Harcourt Brace Janovich, Fort Worth.

Stern P.N. (1994) Eroding grounded theory. In: *Critical Issues in Qualitative Research Methods* (ed. J.M. Morse), pp. 212–223, Sage, Thousand Oaks, California.

Strauss A. & Corbin J. (1990) *Basics of Qualitative Research: Grounded Theory Procedures and Techniques*. Sage, Newbury Park, California.

Strauss A. & Corbin J. (1994) Grounded theory methodology: an overview. In: *The Handbook of Qualitative Research* (eds N.K. Denzin & Y. Lincoln), pp. 173–285, Sage, Thousand Oaks, California.

Strauss A.L., Schatzman L., Bucher R., Ehrlich D. & Sabshin M. (1964) *Psychiatric Ideologies and Institutions*. Transaction Books, New Brunswick.

Swanson J.M. (1986) The formal qualitative interview for grounded theory. In: *From Practice to Grounded Theory; Qualitative Research in Nursing* (eds W.C. Chenitz & J.M. Swanson), pp. 66–78, Addison-Wesley, Menlo Park, California.

Tesch R. (1991) Software for qualitative researchers. In: *Using Computers in Qualitative Research* (eds N.G. Fielding & R.M. Lee), pp. 16–37, Sage, London.

Thompson N. (1995) *Theory and Practice in Health and Social Care*. Open University Press, Milton Keynes.

Truzzi M. (1974) *Verstehen: Subjective Understanding in the Social Sciences*. Addison-Wesley, Reading, Massachusetts.

Ward R. (1990) Meeting points. *Nursing Times*, 86 (22), 58–60.

Wilde V. (1992) Controversial hypotheses on the relationship between researcher and informant in qualitative research. *Journal of Advanced Nursing*, 17, 234–242.

Chapter 2

Initial Steps in the Research Process

This chapter will cover:

- The selection and formulation of the research question
- The literature review
- Writing a research proposal
- Access and entry to the setting

Nurses who wish to do research go through a process of selecting the research topic and defining the research question. They must make sure that they have a sound design, and that this design fits the chosen topic. Although the initial steps in different types of research are similar, qualitative researchers use the principles and language of qualitative enquiry, as Cresswell (1994:2) states:

> 'This study is defined as an enquiry process of understanding a social or human problem, based on building a complex, holistic picture, formed with words, reporting detailed views of informants, and conducted in a natural setting'.

Selecting and formulating the research question

The first step in the process is the selection of the research question or topic. Nurses and midwives often notice problems in their work setting which, they feel, need investigation so that solutions or remedies for unsatisfactory situations or behaviour might be found. Sometimes the topic emerges from the literature linked to a particular area of professional work where gaps in knowledge can be identified. Research studies fill these gaps in existing knowledge and enhance understanding. For nurses and midwives understanding is not always enough; they also seek solutions to problems in the clinical setting. Brink & Wood (1988:2) describe the essence of a research question: 'A research question is an explicit query about a problem or issue that can be challenged, examined and analysed and that will yield useful new information'.

Personal observation and experience, as well as discussion with others, guide individuals towards the topic for research. Events and interactions often provide nurses and midwives with an interest or a puzzle and generate the wish to know more. The research question is a statement about what they want to find out and stems directly from a problem experienced in the clinical area or in their personal and professional lives.

It is important that the problem is related to the nurses' work; for instance, if they are working in the field of paediatrics it would be inappropriate for them to undertake a project with old people, however much it might arouse their interest. One of our students, for example, a paediatric nurse and clinical tutor, chose to examine the childhood experience of asthma because of her involvement with children who have this condition (Ireland, 1993). Another student, a member of a management team, studied nurses' views of staff appraisal (Easton, 1995).

Certain criteria should be considered when identifying a research problem:

- It must be researchable
- It must be relevant
- It must be feasible within the allocated time span and resources
- It should be interesting to the researcher

The question must be researchable

Nurses are often confronted with an important ethical or philosophical dilemma which cannot be solved through research. A moral or philosophical question is not researchable; for instance, the question of whether nurses should become involved in euthanasia is answerable only in philosophical but not in research terms. Although the problem need not be a practical one, it must nevertheless result in findings and outcomes. The topic of nurses' perceptions of euthanasia, for instance, would be researchable. 'Do' and 'should' questions are difficult to answer other than with a yes or no. 'Do new mothers have feelings of inadequacy?' would become 'What are the feelings of new mothers about coping with their babies?' to transform it into a research question.

> ## Examples of researchable questions
>
> What is the effect of placing patients in a mixed sex ward? What are staff nurses' perceptions (or experiences) of staff appraisal? How do people with multiple sclerosis cope with their illness?

The topic should be relevant

This means that the topic is usually linked to clinical practice or professional issues. The question might be important for other health professionals too, and for society in general, and the answer will advance theoretical nursing and midwifery knowledge. The results should be applicable to practice, education or management, legitimising existing practices or leading the way towards change. Beginners, however, such as pre-registration students, might well take on a simple study suitable for showing that they understand the research process and can produce a valid and useful project. We advise novice researchers not to undertake research involving patients except in exceptional circumstances, for instance if they have long nursing experience, special expertise in their field and have expert supervision. The problem is that patients often find it easier to talk to the junior nurses, and the latter tend to gather more 'quotable' data than senior nurses.

The work must be feasible

Nurses are sometimes over-ambitious, especially if they are beginning researchers. Rather than reflecting on the time the study may take, some of the detailed procedures and the complexity of analysis, they want to start the study straight away, before they have a thorough knowledge of methodology. Lack of time can become a problem in qualitative research because transcribing, coding and categorising data stretches over a long period. A simple small scale study using a well documented research strategy is far less time consuming than a complex piece of triangulation.

The research should be feasible in terms of resources and accessibility of participants, and researchers should identify whose resources will be used. The topic might be inappropriate because of major ethical and access problems which cannot be overcome, such as superiors not giving permission to do the research or patients' vulnerability. The research needs also to be feasible in terms of participant numbers or availability. Last but not least, it must be within the researcher's knowledge and capability. To novice researchers we give the advice to be clear and straightforward. The clearer the question, the clearer the outcome of the study.

The topic should be of interest to the researcher

If the topic is interesting, it can stimulate and motivate rather than generate boredom after a short time into the study. The storyline of the project is not merely controlled by the participants but it reflects the interest of the researcher. The selection of the focus takes time, reflection and discussion with others who have knowledge in the field of study. Students in particular should discuss the focus of their work with their tutors and supervisors. All too often, new researchers in qualitative research choose a question which is designed to deal with factual issues and needs a survey rather than a qualitative approach.

> Example
>
> A nurse decides to research the availability of community services in the area. He or she questions patients and nurses in the community about access to services. A qualitative study would not be useful, as a survey questionnaire is more appropriate to elicit this detailed information about facts.

Quantitative researchers focus on a very specific area, while qualitative researchers initially formulate the question in more general terms. Indeed, the research design develops and changes, it is not fully developed from the outset but evolutionary rather than strictly defined. This needs flexibility on the part of researchers. They cannot plan exactly what they do because they need to respond to participants and events during the research process. This means that precise objectives can rarely be written before the start. The qualitative researcher generally begins with a broad question in the data collection and becomes more specific in the process of the research (progressive focusing).

Example

A community nurse might be interested in the experience of informal carers of ill or disabled people. As many of her clients are elderly patients with arthritis, she decides that the focus of the study should be the experience of relatives who look after old people with arthritis. However, on searching the literature on this topic, she finds that a large number of studies exist about daughters caring for their elderly arthritic relatives, but nobody has yet looked at spouse carers. The final aim of the project then is 'to explore the caring experience of people who look after an elderly spouse with arthritis'.

Reviewing the literature

After identifying the research question, investigators review the literature consisting of all the information published and closely related to the area of the project. Included are both primary and secondary sources. Primary sources are produced by those who developed original work on a subject or researched this topic, while secondary information is merely a report, summary or reference to original work.

Researchers review the literature for the following reasons:

- To find out what is already known about the subject and identify gaps in knowledge
- To describe how the study contributes to existing knowledge of a topic area
- To avoid duplicating other people's work

Although replication is sometimes the intention of quantitative projects, qualitative researchers realise that their studies can never be truly replicated because this type of research depends on the unique researcher–participant relationship.

Through reading reports, researchers can identify what knowledge about the subject of their study already exists, the way in which it was generated and the methods that were adopted. They may find a large number of studies on the particular topic and decide to avoid it, not wishing to focus on issues which others have thoroughly examined at an earlier stage. There is little justification for researchers keeping to their original ideas if the topic has already been addressed exhaustively and adequately elsewhere. However, the literature sometimes points to problems within the subject area which have not yet been investigated.

Example

One of our students works in a community hospital. She was particularly interested in how patients viewed the hospital. She found that patients' perceptions relating to small local hospitals had been studied in the USA, but that there were no data from Britain. This was the gap she identified (undergraduate student experience).

The use of literature in qualitative research

Currently there is a debate about the place of the literature in qualitative research. We know that in quantitative studies researchers read the literature about a topic area and give a detailed report in the literature review before they start the field-work. In the early days of qualitative investigations, researchers were encouraged to start without a literature review so that they would not be directed in their research, as it was believed that a detailed review would invalidate the qualitative research study. Indeed, Glaser (1978, 1992) strongly advises against any type of literature review. However, Morse (1994a) warns us of the folly of trying to 're-invent the wheel', because an answer to the question may already exist.

In any case, a researcher's mind is not a *tabula rasa*, especially not when reaching the thesis stage (Glaser & Strauss, 1967; Morse, 1994a). Although it is inappropriate to start with a fully developed theoretical model and an in-depth literature review, there is a danger in starting without any prior idea of what has already been done in the field. The introductory literature review (or overview) should not be seen to lead to *a priori* assumptions or the researchers could be accused of contaminating the data or their own interpretation (Morse, 1994b).

Researchers do not enter the study with a fixed framework (Minichiello *et al.*, 1990), nor have they identified hypotheses or fully developed theories for their research as do many quantitative researchers. However, in qualitative research a conceptual framework is necessary too, as the study must be linked to other research and ideas about the topic. An overview of the literature often takes place prior to the study, but the literature search and review is ongoing. The literature becomes another source for data in the main body of the study, where it is guided by the emerging categories (Chenitz, 1986). The researchers compare or contrast their own findings with those of other studies and engage in an active debate, about results reported in the literature. This happens throughout the study.

Often, a category or construct that researchers discover and develop is reflected in other disciplines or areas of knowledge. They can then follow up ideas about the emerging concept in the literature. A look at the nursing literature does not always suffice; psychological or sociological literature might also be useful.

> ## Example
>
> An investigator finds that 'returning to normal' is a major issue for people who have had a myocardial infarction. He or she then follows up the idea of 'becoming normal, being normal, normalisation' etc., in other fields of study. The research in other studies about people with a disability or another illness condition, and how they try to achieve normality, can then become part of the data in the study of patients with myocardial infarction.

Practicalities

Many researchers summarise research studies from the literature, and the major concepts involved, on cards which they file alphabetically from the beginning of their research. This way they can access the ideas and topic areas more quickly when they want them at a later stage.

If strong factual claims are made in the introduction or literature review (for instance 'Recent research has shown . . .', or 'Some nurse researchers suggest . . .') they must be substantiated with names, and evidence should be given.

Writing a research proposal

This is sometimes called the *research protocol*; the term *proposal* is generally used in an academic setting.

Before starting the data collection, researchers write a proposal – a detailed summary of what they will be examining, why they adopt the particular research focus, and how they will proceed. The proposal is intended to clarify the research for submission to ethics committees, funding agencies, official gatekeepers such as managers and, for student work, to supervisors. The proposal is a detailed plan of action which has to convince the reader that the researcher knows enough to undertake the project.

The proposal consists of the following main elements:

(1) *Abstract*
(2) *Introduction*
  - Problem statement and rationale (justification for the study)
  - The aim of the research
(3) *Brief discussion of the relevant literature*
  - A discussion of other researchers' work which demonstrates the need for this particular study
(4) *Methodology*
  - Theoretical basis and justification of the methodology
  - Sample selection and sampling procedures
  - Context and setting

- Data collection and strategies
- Data analysis
- Ethical and entry issues

(5)   Timetable and costing

(6)   Dissemination

Researchers generally proceed in this order, although reviewers (supervisors, ethics committees or funding bodies) might have their own format for the proposal. Proposals for most types of research are similar, although qualitative researchers do not follow rigidly a pre-planned path but adopt more pragmatic procedures (Wilson, 1985). This might mean change and reformulation at a later stage during the process. Sandelowski *et al.* (1989) too, remind qualitative researchers that the proposal is the beginning of a developing design which cannot be fixed and rigid in qualitative enquiry. We advise inexperienced researchers, however, to follow clearly structured, conventional guidelines.

Abstract

The abstract in the research proposal is a brief summary of the aim, methods and reasons why the research will be done.

Introduction

This section sets the scene for the research and must be clear and precise. Readers can only understand the proposal in context. In the introduction researchers demonstrate quality and feasibility of the study and the reasons for it.

The problem statement and rationale

Nurses briefly describe the research focus, the way in which they became aware of the problem, and why they want to find out about it. They describe the context in which it takes place. It is important that the research problem is not trivial but has significance for nursing. The potential usefulness of the project for the profession might be explained. Researchers can address a new problem which occurred in the setting or adopt a new approach to a familiar problem. They demonstrate the significance of the work by explaining why the research is important, and/or how it could possibly help in improving nursing or midwifery practice. Research funded by the National Health Service or related funding agencies must identify potential benefits to the NHS.

The rationale gives the reasons for the research, which have often emerged through observation of a problem in a particular situation or were stimulated by reading about an event, a crisis or question in the clinical or community setting. At this stage researchers can mention some of the claims and suggestions that other writers make about the topic or area of study. The investigation of the problem should fill a gap in professional knowledge, however small that gap may be. Stern (1985) suggests that qualitative research is particularly appropriate when little is known about the area of research, because the researcher does not start with pre-conceived ideas.

The aim

The aim of the study – a statement of the researcher's intentions – is made explicit. A broad statement of the aim is sufficient although some researchers give a general aim and a series of more specific objectives or steps to reach this aim. We would advise against specific objectives as they might rigidify the study by directing it from the outset rather than being guided by the ideas of the participants. If objectives are given, the researcher must be prepared to change them in the course of the research. The overarching aim is usually concerned with an understanding of participants' feelings, experiences and perceptions as they have developed in the setting and context.

Examples of aims

The aim of this study is to explore the experiences of children who suffer from asthma.

The purpose of my study is to describe the perceptions of experienced and new nurses of the expanded role.

The study aims to examine why people with cancer visit alternative practitioners

---

Cresswell (1994) advises qualitative researchers to keep the aim non-directional; not to describe cause and effect but to give a general sense of the main idea using terms such as explore, develop and describe. Generally the statement of the study's aim should not contain more than a maximum of 25 words.

The literature

This is sometimes called the 'initial literature review'. The literature demonstrates the amount and level of knowledge which exists in the area of study. On the basis of an initial scan of relevant studies done by others, the researcher can decide whether to proceed with the work. It is important to mention not only seminal studies on the subject if they exist, but also include the most recent.

In a qualitative literature overview the discussion of the literature tends to be more limited than in other types of research. As the data have primacy, qualitative researchers tend to avoid taking too much direction from the literature, and in consequence they only discuss a few major research studies. We would like to remind students, however, that the literature will become part of the data and the data analysis at a later stage. This is discussed earlier in this chapter, in the section on literature.

The methodology

As stated before, methodology is concerned with the ideas and principles on which procedures are based. Methods consist of the procedures and strategies rooted in a methodology. Students must identify, describe and justify the methodology they adopt and the strategies and procedures involved. It is, of course, important that the methods fit the research question. It must be remembered that some of the details of a qualitative research project cannot be pre-specified as they arise during the research process. The access to the participants and the initial sample size must be explained as well as other sampling procedures. An explanation of purposive and theoretical sampling is given. At this stage researchers describe the type of inter-view or observation and the setting in which it takes place. Finally, the data analysis is described in a few paragraphs with examples for each step.

Limitations of the study

Researchers list the constraints and limitations of the study, and how they would overcome them. Limitations are weaknesses in the research. By stating these and solutions to them, researchers show their careful preparation for the study. For example, one of the limitations of qualitative research is the lack of generalisability, which must be acknowledged. When stating the limitations researchers must suggest ways to overcome them. It can be explained, for instance, how the lack of generalisability need not be a problem by describing attempts to achieve typicality or specificity.

Example

A researcher planned a study researching students' learning of the role of the midwife. She intended to do this in her own university, in a department of health studies, through in-depth interviewing of students and mentors. She realised that the outcome of the study would only be related to her own setting and could not be generalised. To achieve typicality, she studied three other settings in different areas of the country. Important similarities in the different settings have already been found. When this study is finished, it might well show that the results show typicality, meaning that they are typical not only for one setting, but across similar settings (post-graduate student experience).

Entry and ethical issues should be considered at this stage in one or two paragraphs. (This is discussed in the section on access in this chapter and in Chapter 3.)

Dissemination

Researchers identify the readership for whom they write and explain the usefulness of the study for the particular group they address. They can state how they will disseminate the results of the study, be it through journals, books or other media, such as conferences, video and audio tapes.

Timetable and resources

Reviewers wish to see a timetable for the research to become convinced of its feasibility. Therefore qualitative researchers submit a projected work schedule for the research even though they cannot always predict how long exactly each step is going to take. Each step is recorded on the time line. This time line can be written or drawn as a diagram. It must be remembered that *the analysis of data in qualitative research takes a long time*. The literature has to be searched after the identification of major categories and built into the findings and discussion. The write-up is revised until a storyline is clearly discernible. All this takes time.

Example of a time frame for an undergraduate student project

June/July
Initial literature review and formulation of research question
Gaining approval from gatekeepers, ethics committee and participants
Writing proposal
August/September
Data collection (for instance, interviewing and participant observation)
Start of analysis (coding and categorising)
September – January
Further data collection and analysis
Literature review related to emerging categories
Final decision on categories and major themes
January–March
Writing up

This could also be presented in diagrammatic form.

It must be made clear that data collection and analysis proceed at the same time and interact, and that there is an ongoing process of searching the literature which is linked to the emerging categories. Researchers specify the use of resources and other costs to demonstrate that the research can be adequately funded. Resourcing and costs are of major importance in proposals for grant-giving bodies and must be detailed. These include clerical costs, paper, computer, letters and mailing, as well as the researcher's time.

It is a good idea to look at one's own proposal in the light of an evaluation checklist. We have added an example below.

Evaluation of a qualitative research proposal

(1) The aim
   (a) Is the aim linked to the discovery of feelings, perceptions and concepts rather than facts?

(b) Is the aim clearly and precisely stated?

(2) Methodology and methods
   (a) Is the methodology justified?
   (b) Does the researcher show an understanding of qualitative enquiry?
   (c) Are the methods, techniques and strategies clearly described in detail (this would include the data collection and analysis)?
   (d) Are the methods appropriate for the problem or topic under study?

(3) The sample
   (a) Does the researcher show how he or she will gain access to the sample?
   (b) Is there an explanation of purposive and/or theoretical sampling?
   (c) Does the researcher describe the essential features of the sample?

(4) The literature
   (a) Has a gap in knowledge been identified through an initial literature review?
   (b) Does the researcher state that the literature will be integrated into the discussion and become part of the data?

(5) Ethical issues
   (a) Have the major ethical issues been taken into consideration?
   (b) Has permission been sought from the participants and the relevant gatekeepers including ethics committees?
   (c) Will the researcher guarantee anonymity to the participants and the right to withdraw at any time?

(6) Practical issues
   (a) Is the topic area researchable and feasible?
   (b) Does the researcher have enough time to undertake the study?
   (c) Are the resources sufficient for the proposed project?

(7) Application to nursing or midwifery
   (a) Are there any implications for clinical practice, nurse education or nursing management?
   (b) Will the outcome of the study have potenttial benefits for the participants?

Access and entry

Nursing and midwifery researchers, be they experienced or students, must ask permission for entry to the setting and access to the participants. Gaining access means that they can observe the situation, talk to members in the setting, read the necessary documents and interview potential participants. Formal permission is important in any research and protects both researchers and participants. Access is sought in various ways. Some nurse researchers put up a notice on a public board in the hospital in which they work. Others ask permission from a self-help group, such as a group of carers, to talk to the members and ask them whether they wish to participate. Price (1993) recruited her sample via diabetes newsletters which were distributed in an area. There are a number of ways to access potential informants, but voluntary participation must be ensured.

The choice of setting

Researchers search for an appropriate setting. The location where the research takes place must be suitable. For this the researcher has to know the setting intimately, and for nurses who research their own setting it is not difficult. There is, of course, a very important difference between knowledge of, say, a paediatric oncology setting in general and of researching it on the particular unit in which the nurse works. Jorgensen (1989) claims that if much is known about the setting, it is easier to find out whether the study is feasible in its proposed form. Some settings are inappropriate for the particular research question. There is no point in planning an ambitious study if access to the setting proves impossible.

Hitchcock & Hughes (1989) give guidelines in the entry process and advise the researcher to:

- establish points of contact
- describe the aims and scope of the project
- anticipate sensitive aspects of the research
- be aware of and sensitive to the organisational hierarchy in the setting
- be conscious of the effects of change through research

First then, nurses need to make contact with people in the setting who can give permission for access and with those whom they wish to observe and interview.

Second, the nurse explains early and clearly the type of project and its scope and aims. It must be remembered, however, that the explanation cannot be too detailed as the research might be prejudiced if all the issues are explained at this early stage, and participants would be guided too firmly towards certain issues rather than giving their own ideas and perceptions to the researcher.

Third, sensitive areas for research and vulnerable people must be treated with thoughtfulness and care.

Fourth, the researcher must be aware of the hierarchy in the system and know that conflicts between the interests of those at the top and those at the bottom of the hierarchy may exist. All individual participants involved should, of course, be asked for permission to undertake the study.

Fifth, the researcher might have an effect on the setting. This may not only be threatening to the people involved but could also skew the research. This threat can be diminished if the researcher gets to know the people in the setting and establishes a relationship of trust.

Access to gatekeepers

Researchers negotiate with the *gatekeepers*, the people who have the power to grant or withhold access. There may be a number of these at different places in the hierarchy of the organisation. Researchers should not just ask the person directly in charge but also others who hold the power to start and stop the research. This includes managers, clinicians, consultants, GPs or other personnel whose patients or clients might be observed or interviewed. For instance, if a nurse wishes to observe interaction on a ward, he or she must not only ask the consent of the manager of the Trust and the local ethics committee, but also that of the ward manager, the people working on the ward and, most importantly, the patients involved.

All gatekeepers have power and control of access, but those at the top of the hierarchy are the most powerful and should be asked first because they can restrict access even if everybody else agrees. If they cooperate, the path of the research can be smoothed, and their recommendations might make others more willing to collaborate. Figure 2.1 gives an example of an ethical submission form.

There can also be problems with gatekeepers: they might make demands that the researchers cannot fulfil, trying to guide them in a particular direction or denying access to some individuals. Often their knowledge of research is based on familiarity with randomised controlled trials or surveys; hence the nature of qualitative research and the aims and objectives of the study must be explained. The topic might have to be negotiated to fit in with the social organisation, physical environment or timetable of the setting. Researchers cannot start without permission and must take the wishes of the gatekeepers into account; it is important, however, that they are not seen by the participants as a tool of management because this would affect the data.

Usually gatekeepers do not interfere in the research process, though ethics committees can and do. In research carried out with financial and social support from superiors, there is sometimes a danger that gatekeepers have their own expectations and sometimes attempt to manipulate the research, intentionally or unintentionally. This can affect the researchers' direction or report of the work, and they might find that they are influenced by these expectations. As gatekeepers are in a position of power over the researcher, resistance might be difficult.

Example

An experienced nurse intended to interview patients with a serious condition about their need for counselling as part of an undergraduate study. His immediate superior not only encouraged the research, she also saw it as important because of the support that might be given to future patients with the same condition. The ethics committee had given its approval. However, one of the consultants on the ward disagreed with the form of the proposed research and refused permission for interviews of the patients in his care.

A series of complications and difficulties followed. On the one hand the research was seen as important by the researcher and his colleagues. On the other, to go ahead meant directly contravening the consultant's wishes and

> Example *contd.*
>
> generating conflict between him and the researcher's superiors. Endless debates and discussions would waste precious time, and in the end the researcher decided to explore the perceptions of the nurses who cared for the patients instead of interviewing the patients (undergraduate student experience).

Although the piece of research did not directly explore the feelings of patients, it produced results which helped in their care and avoided conflict on the ward. This example shows that powerful people within the setting can generate difficulties for the researcher who often has to compromise.

The new contract arrangements between purchasers and providers in the reformed National Health Service (Ham, 1991) could also lead to more constraints on researchers as institutional objectives might take precedence over individual research interest because of the prioritising of resources. Staff time costs money.

Researchers are denied access for a variety of reasons:

- The researcher is seen as unsuitable by gatekeepers
- It is feared that an observer might disturb the setting
- There is suspicion and fear of criticism
- Sensitive issues are being investigated
- Potential participants in the research may be embarrassed or fearful

Powerful gatekeepers might see researchers as unsuitable because of gender, age or lack of trustworthiness. They must be convinced that the researcher is able to cope with the study and trustworthy. Friends and acquaintances who are already involved in the researcher's chosen location can sometimes persuade those in power of the ability and trustworthiness of the researcher. If researchers are very young, the gatekeepers might feel that they lack credibility. Some female writers such as Gurney (1991) have felt that they were not taken seriously by male informants in a position of power. On the other hand, Gurney felt that occasionally females are seen as less threatening, especially in a male dominated environment.

Managers might deny access if they feel that the setting will be disturbed by the presence of the researcher. A ward climate might change because everybody feels that he or she watches every task and movement that occurs; therefore it is important that observers and interviewers immerse themselves in the setting until they become part of it and do not create an 'observer effect'.

Ethics committees

Ethics committees would have to scrutinise any research project which involves patients/clients or their relatives. Ramos (1989) suggests that standard research ethics cannot always be applied in qualitative approaches. It would be difficult to

Organization/Department _____

ETHICAL SUBMISSION (UNDERGRADUATE PROJECTS)
please type or print

Name of student

Professional/Academic qualifications (if any)

Course

Title of study

Aim of study

Method
(Please underline those which apply and supply *brief* supplementary details where required – no more than one page)

Questionnaire   *Standardised interviews*   *In-depth interviews*

Please attach draft copies of questionnaires/schedules, or attach brief outline of the type of questioning which will be used.

Observation studies

Please specify if video/tape recorders are to be used, and outline how observations will be recorded. If physical observations are to be made, please specify how these will be obtained. Please attach these details.

Intervention/experimental studies

Please attach details of all interventions and control procedures. Identify measurements to be used.

Other Please provide details.

Fig. 2.1 Example of an ethical submission form (initially developed by Walker in 1991).

(1) How large is your sample size?

(2) Who will the participants be?

(3) How will you recruit the participants?

(4) Describe how participants will be informed of the purpose of the study

Attach draft information sheet where appropriate.

(5) How will consent be obtained (e.g. in writing or verbal) and what steps will you take to avoid coercion?

Attach draft consent form where appropriate.

(6) What steps will you take to protect participants from any possible physical or psychological harm?

(7) What steps will you take to protect confidentiality and anonymity?

(8) Which hospitals/units/sites/settings will be involved?

(9) Will your study involve the time of staff members in the above locations? If so, please estimate how much.

(10) Please itemise all costs and state who will fund these. (Please include all photocopying, postage, work time for yourself and others.)

(11) Permission must be obtained from managers, clinicians, GPs and/or other relevant personnel. Please ask them to indicate this by signing below:

Name	Signature	Designation

Student: Please sign below to verify that these are the full details of the study.

Names, designations and signatures of supervisor(s)

Name _____	Name _____
Designation _____	Designation _____
Signature _____	Signature _____

All changes must be notified to your supervisors and resubmitted if necessary

identify a single set of rules for all research because of its variety, although the principles are similar for different types of research and for most settings and situations.

An ethics submission form is filled out when researching patients or clients. This includes the name, position and location of the researcher, the title and aim of the study, the sampling and research methods, the number of participants and the way in which they will be asked for consent. The form is sent to the ethics committee for approval. If it does not meet with approval it must be resubmitted until it has passed the committee as the research cannot start without approval. For research with clients, it does not suffice to gain permission from immediate superiors, managers, consultants or GPs. Any piece of research that deals with sensitive issues should have approval from the ethics committee, even if it researches colleagues rather than clients.

Ramos (1989) claims that not all health professionals have had formal instruction in the ethics of qualitative research, and members of committees are not always aware of the complex issues and dilemmas in these methods. They are used to proposals in the field of biomedical research or quantitative surveys with large numbers of respondents and random sampling. For the qualitative researcher this means clear presentation of ethics forms and a detailed statement of methods and procedures to the committee. Sometimes the committee demands a questionnaire. The qualitative researcher must then send an interview guide with the type of questions that might be asked. Ethics committees can call on researchers to explain and defend their research.

Access to participants

Researchers ask potential participants for permission to interview or observe, stating clearly the right to refusal or withdrawal and assuring confidentiality. In research with children, the consent of parents and of the children themselves must be obtained. If researchers are not known to potential participants, they introduce themselves by name and identify their institution. It is useful to carry a short letter of introduction from the institution.

Consent forms are given or sent to participants for signature. The form gives the aim and outline of the research and describes briefly the implications for the informants. The consent form should not be too long and must be clearly expressed in plain English, not in technical terminology or jargon. The signing of a consent form is not universally practised, and many participants give their verbal consent. In circumstances where written consent is unduly difficult to obtain or intrusive, researchers do not always ask for it. Written consent may, in fact, prejudice the study or interfere with the researcher–participant relationship by formalising it. In researching colleagues too, the written consent form is often seen as unnecessary. However, students must be aware that some ethics committees insist on a consent form.

This section is further developed in Chapter 3.

When the main steps have been taken, the research can begin, always taking into account appropriate timing, site and situation.

Summary

The first step in the process is selection of the research topic and focus. This is often based on experience of a problem in the clinical area, and occasionally on personal experience or the professional literature.

After an initial short overview of previous research the researcher identifies the gaps in knowledge; the specific topic area and methodology should be appropriate for the topic.

Following ethical guidelines, the researcher then writes a research proposal and seeks access to gatekeepers and participants. It is essential that research on patients and clients, or other sensitive research, is vetted by the local ethics committee.

References

Brink P.J. & Wood M.J. (1988) *Basic Steps in Planning Nursing Research*. Jones and Bartlett, Boston.

Chenitz W.C. (1986) Getting started: the research proposal for a grounded theory study. In *From Practice to Grounded Theory: Qualitative Research in Nursing* (eds W.C. Chenitz & J.M. Swanson), pp. 39–47, Addison-Wesley, Menlo Park, California.

Cresswell J.W. (1994) *Research Design: Qualitative and Quantitative Approaches*. Sage, Thousand Oaks, California.

Easton D. (1995) Nurses' views of staff appraisal. Unpublished BSc project, Bournemouth University, Bournemouth.

Glaser B.G. (1978) *Theoretical Sensitivity*. Sociology Press, Mill Valley, California.

Glaser B.G. (1992) *Basics of Grounded Theory Analysis*. Sociology Press, Mill Valley, California.

Glaser B.G. & Strauss A.L. (1967) *The Discovery of Grounded Theory: Strategies for Qualitative Research*. Aldine De Gruyter, New York.

Gurney J.N. (1991) Female researchers in male-dominated settings: implications for short-term versus long-term research. In *Experiencing Fieldwork: An Inside View of Qualitative Research* (eds W.B. Shaffir & R.A. Stebbins), pp. 53–61, Sage, Newbury Park, California.

Ham, C. (1991) *The New National Health Service*. Radcliffe Medical Press, Oxford.

Hitchcock G. & Hughes D. (1989) *Research and the Teacher: A Qualitative Introduction to School-Based Research*. Routledge, London.

Ireland L.M. (1993) Establishing normality: the childhood experience of asthma. Unpublished BSc research project, Bournemouth University, Bournemouth.

Jorgensen D.L. (1989) *Participant Observation*. Sage, Newbury Park, California.

Minichiello V., Aroni R., Timewell E. & Alexander L. (1990) *In-Depth Interviewing: Researching People*. Longman Cheshire, Melbourne.

Morse J.M. (1994a) Editorial: Going in 'blind'. *Qualitative Health Research*, 4(1), 3–5.

Morse J.M. (1994b) Emerging from the data: the cognitive process of analysis in qualitative inquiry. In *Critical Issues in Qualitative Research Methods* (ed. J.M. Morse), pp. 23–43, Sage, Thousand Oaks, California.

Price M. (1993) An experiential model of learning diabetes self-management. *Qualitative Health Research*, 3(1), 29–54.

Ramos M.C. (1989) Some ethical implications of qualitative research. *Research in Nursing and Health*, **12**, 57–63.

Sandelowski M., Davies D.H. & Harris B.G. (1989) Artful design: writing a proposal in the natural paradigm. *Research in Nursing and Health*, **12**, 77–84.

Stern P.N. (1985) Using grounded theory in nursing research. In *Qualitative Research Methods in Nursing* (ed. M. Leininger), pp. 149–160, W.B. Saunders, Philadelphia.

Wilson H.S. (1985) Research proposal: the practical imagination at work. *The Journal of Nursing Administration*, **15**(2), 5–7.

In this chapter we will examine the following:

- The basic ethical framework applied to research
- Ethical problems and considerations
- Practical solutions to ethical problems

Access and entry are discussed in the preceding chapter.

Ethical issues have to be considered in all research methods, be they quantitative or qualitative. Researchers apply the principles which protect the participants in the research from harm or risk and follow professional and legal rules which are laid down in the code of professional conduct (UKCC, 1992) and research guidelines. Nurses and midwives have to justify the research not only to ethics and research committees but also to superiors, gatekeepers and research participants. They must recognise the right of informants to refuse participation in the project or to withdraw from it if they wish. Couchman & Dawson (1995) state that the rights of the individual are: not to be harmed, informed consent, voluntary participation, confidentiality, anonymity, dignity and self-respect. These rights can be set within the four principles outlined by Beauchamp & Childress (1994):

- The principle of respect for autonomy
- The principle of non-maleficence (doing no harm)
- The principle of beneficence (doing good)
- The principle of justice

Respect for autonomy means that the participants in the research must make a free, independent and informed choice without coercion. The good derived from the research must be weighed against the potential harm, and the benefits must outweigh the risks for the individual and the wider society. The principle of justice implies that the research strategies and procedures are fair and just.

Historically, attempts at establishing international rules for ethical research stem from the time after World War II, as a result of the criminal trials in Germany. The *Nuremberg Code* contained guidelines for consent and discontinuation of studies and advised on the balance between risks and benefits. Most of these rules were concerned with experimental research. The *Declaration of Helsinki* (World Medical Association, 1964, revised 1975) differentiates between therapeutic research (to explore the effects of new treatments) and non-therapeutic research (to discover new knowledge).

The basic ethical framework for nursing research

To appreciate specific features of ethics in qualitative research it is important to understand the philosophical assumptions on which they are based. This chapter addresses the branch of philosophy concerning value in focusing on ethical issues in qualitative research. Ethics originates from the Greek word 'ethos' meaning character (Tschudin, 1986) and refers to both individual character and ways of behaving. There are two approaches in ethics, the normative approach (what we should do) and the descriptive approach (what we actually do).

Nursing and midwifery ethics take primarily the normative approach which is concerned with guiding professionals to 'safeguard the interest and well-being of patients and clients' (UKCC, 1992). In order to achieve this, researchers need sufficient background in professional studies which focus on ethical and legal aspects of the professional–client relationship. Therefore, more than information about ethical codes is required. The researcher needs to draw on the ethical theories and principles in research in order to resolve ethical dilemmas. Whilst Clarke (1991) demonstrates the use of codes in health research, Tschudin (1992:64) argues that codes 'point to what should be'. Beauchamp & Childress (1994) provide a simple, linear model to establish where actions, theories, principles and codes fit in the process of ethical decision making. Principles are rooted in theories of ethics and generate rules on which researchers base their specific judgments and behaviour. The model evolves in the following way: ethical theories – principles – rules – particular judgments and actions.

This model is best explained by discussing moral theory. Moral theory which informs ethical decision-making can be divided into two major categories, non-consequentialist and consequentialist. Deontological theory (from the Greek work 'deon' meaning duty) is often referred to as non-consequentialist. This is due to the fact that decisions for actions and judgments are not based solely on the consequences of that action or judgment.

One of the originators of this theory is the German philosopher Immanuel Kant (1724–1804) who set out to investigate the possibility of metaphysical thought, that is, the knowledge of the existence of God and the immortality of the soul, and also whether human beings have free will. Kant developed his now famous supreme moral law which he saw as a law for all. A major tenet of this law is that no person should be treated merely as a means but always as an end. Ethical decisions are based on belief in moral law. Nursing and midwifery research based on these ideas should take into account the ways and means of achieving the aims of the research and its meaning for individuals.

In contrast to these ideas, consequential ethical theory (or utilitarianism) places more emphasis on the consequences of actions. Beauchamp & Childress (1994) show that utility means usefulness. This theory claims that that which is right is also most useful. Prominent in the development of utilitarian theories of ethics was the British philosopher John Stuart Mill (1806–1873). However, the principle of utility originated from Jeremy Bentham (1748–1832) who disseminated the idea that 'the greatest happiness of the greatest number' is the main goal of social ethics and a criterion for morality. Mill developed this principle into a moral theory arguing that actions are right if they promote happiness, and wrong if they bring about the reverse of happiness.

In essence then, utilitarianism attempts to promote the idea of the greatest happiness for the greatest number, which is the principle of utility. In terms of nursing and midwifery research this would mean that the consequences of the research and its positive outcome for the greatest number of clients is the important focus.

Deontological and utilitarian differences can produce practical disagreements. Beauchamp & Childress (1994) show throughout their work that deontologists can often be sceptical of research that might potentially violate certain rights, like respect for autonomy and protection against harm. Utilitarians, on the other hand, tend to support research of all types which involves human beings, because its social benefits are paramount. Yet the protagonists of the different approaches usually agree that the ethical stance in research should take account of theories, principles and codes of ethics.

Rules and professional codes form the third tier in the model. Rules of veracity (truth telling) make lying to and deception of the research participants wrong. Other established rules are concerned with privacy and confidentiality, which have been discussed before, and fidelity (faithfulness). Beauchamp & Childress (1994) set these rules within the professional–client relationship and see them as very important for any research. Nurses and midwives, of course, draw on these rules to form their code of professional conduct (UKCC, 1992). However, ethical codes can only provide guidelines for behaviour and are themselves based on ethical principles and theories. This brings us back to the model in its entirety.

Robinson & Thorne (1988) outline the dilemma of ethics in relation to qualitative health care research. They suggest four major issues: informed consent, influence, immersion and intervention. Informed consent is recognised as problematic in qualitative research because data collection and analysis occur simultaneously, and whilst consent may be implied at one stage of the research, it cannot be assumed at another stage when the researcher's objectives change on the basis of the information provided.

Influence in research means a process of changing something whilst studying it. Researchers influence the research and its findings. Qualitative researchers recognise clearly that biases occur and attempt to make these explicit in the report. The researcher as the major data gathering tool must uncover the thought processes which lead to the findings. The findings are then explained within the social and interactional context of the research process. Nurses and midwives must account for the influences of their professional perspectives in the process and outcome of the research.

The third issue mentioned by Robinson & Thorne (1988) refers to immersion. Qualitative research requires the researcher to become immersed in the data. This immersion generates familiarity with the setting, the process and the world of the participants. Through this involvement, a certain amount of subjectivity may occur. As data collection and analysis are taking place at the same time, a measure of objectivity – standing back from the data – is needed. Robinson and Thorne suggest that health professionals engaged in qualitative research have to develop strategies to balance the subjective and objective elements inherent in immersion. They advocate that researchers describe how the tension between these elements was managed.

Intervention is perhaps the most contentious dilemma in qualitative research. The issue concerns the reality of the health professionals' clinical roles. Most research has no immediate result and researchers cannot easily intervene, but the tension between professional and researcher roles still exists.

One of us (S.W.) experienced all these aspects in her research. The following are the issues that arose in the study.

(1) Following ethical approval of the research proposal, individual informed consent was obtained from participating practitioners who reflected on their involvement in some distressing cases of child abuse (identities were not disclosed), which at times caused them to reconsider their participation in the research.

(2) The ethical problem of influence in this study was concerned with the researcher's particular interest and experience in child protection work. It was impossible to 'bracket' out entirely this background. Rather, the aim was to express this as part of the research and make these experiences explicit in the report.,

(3) Immersion of the researcher in the data naturally caused tensions between the lived experiences of the research informants (which could be interpreted subjectively) and the emergence of potential new ideas about communication breakdowns (which could be expressed objectively). To resolve these differing perspectives the researcher had to describe how these were managed in the research process.

(4) Intervention, the term that Robinson & Thorne (1988) suggest, was a contentious issue in this study. The researcher had both a previous practice and management role. Some themes that emerged from the data had immediate implications for current child protection work. Yet ethically it was not appropriate to intervene in practice structures prior to completion of the study and critical analysis of the findings by others.

(5) The implications of these issues for qualitative research mean continuous involvement of both project supervisors and colleagues in the research. Robinson & Thorne (1988) suggest that there should be an ongoing assessment in data gathering with others' monitoring field notes and transcriptions. In student projects this means involvement and advice of the supervisor at all stages of the research.

Ethical problems and considerations

The question of ethics in qualitative health care research is complex and problematic. Qualitative researchers have to consider a variety of issues.

(1) Researchers explore the inner feelings and thoughts of the participants, who are clients, colleagues or other health professionals, and they have to act with sensitivity and diplomacy.

(2) Informed consent is problematic as participants cannot be fully informed at the very beginning because of the tentative and exploratory nature of qualitative research.

(3) The informants' anonymity might be threatened by the detailed description of the research process, the data and the sample.

(4) The vulnerable position of clients and their feelings of obligation might prevent them from refusing participation in the research although they may not wish to do so.

(5) The researcher has conflicting role expectations as investigator and professional.

(6) Participants do not always comprehend the research role of health professionals and see them primarily as carers.

(7) Patients may become fearful and distressed during interviews.

(8) Over-involvement and empathy could create assumptions and inaccuracies in the research.

(8) Ethics committees do not always fully understand the character of qualitative research.

Informed consent and voluntary participation

Informed, voluntary consent is an explicit agreement by the research participants, given without threat or inducement, based on information which any reasonable person would want to receive before consenting to participate (Sieber, 1992).

Qualitative researchers have inherent problems with informed consent. When the research begins they have no specific objectives for the research though they may have general aims or a focus. The nature of qualitative research is its flexibility, the use of unexpected ideas which arise during data collection and the prompts that are allowed during interviews. Qualitative research focuses on the meanings and interpretations of the participants. The researcher develops ideas which are grounded in the data rather than testing previously constructed hypotheses. Therefore, the researcher is not able to inform research participants of the exact path of the research, and informed consent is not a once-and-forever permission but an ongoing process of informed participation (Ford & Reutter, 1990).

The process of informed consent is set firmly within the principle of respect for autonomy. This principle demands that participation is voluntary and that informants are aware not only of the benefits of the research but also of the risks they take. First-time researchers, in particular, should take care that there is no major risk involved, though all research involves some dangers. Participants must be informed throughout about the voluntary nature of participation in research and about the possibility to withdraw at any stage.

It is useful to anticipate potential problems in the course of the research and consider their solutions. The researcher must be aware that the research might

Organisation/Department: _____

CONSENT FORM

Title of study: _____

Researcher's name: _____

Researcher's position (for instance, student nurse, year 3, BSc (Hons)):

_____

Aim of the study: (Give a broad description of the aim of the study)

_____

Interviews will take place with the participants and be tape recorded. Tapes will not be shared by anybody other than the supervisors of the study (and possibly the typist of the transcripts). In the final report of the study examples of the interviews will be given, but these and quotes will remain anonymous; participants will not be recognised because pseudonyms will be used. The participant need not answer any specific questions and can withdraw at any time from the interview or the study.

The researcher will erase the tapes on completion of the project.

This is to show that I (name) _____
consent to participate in the study. I understand that I can withdraw from the study at any time and that I will not be identified in the research report.

Signature of participant: _____

Signature of researcher: _____

Date: _____

Fig. 3.1 Example of a consent form.

threaten participants, superiors or institutions, even if it is intended to have a positive effect. Sim (1991) identifies a major dilemma of researchers: they experience conflict between the recognition of the rights of human beings and the wish to advance professional knowledge.

The researcher should try to be as clear as possible in stating the demands on the time of the participants and about the direction of the research, so that participants can agree or refuse to take part on the basis of this information. Sometimes this might be difficult as the status of a health professional could prevent patients or colleagues from giving honest, open and non-biased answers.

Patients are in a particularly vulnerable position, because they are ill and because of the power relationship with health professionals. Midwives' clients also are in a situation in which they have limited power. Researchers have to weigh the benefits and risks of the research. Health professionals assess the benefits of the project which might help future patients and clients, and they consider the risks involved for research participants.

> **Example**
>
> Consider a nurse who wishes to interview patients with a serious illness about their feelings and the support they receive. The study will almost certainly help in the future because of extended knowledge and information which nurses have gained. Patients, however, may well feel distressed and disturbed by the nurse's probing into private thoughts and feelings at a time when they experience pain, distress and anxiety about their future.

It can be seen that timing is an important issue in qualitative research (Cowles, 1988). Bad timing can inhibit informants, especially when they have recently had a traumatic experience. They might feel threatened at this particular time and too emotionally involved to make rational decisions about taking part in or continuing the research. Qualitative interviews in particular can provoke distressing memories, and the researcher should be prepared to allow the participant to work through this and not abruptly terminate the interview.

> **Example**
>
> A researcher was conducting lengthy interviews in the participants' own homes to find out how they coped with chronic pain. Towards the end, one woman became very upset when she described how her religious faith did not seem strong enough to help her to come to terms with her pain and disability. The researcher, who had no religious affiliation of her own, spent the next three hours persuading the participant that God did not demand perfection. The participant gradually responded positively and was left in a positive frame of mind. Indeed, she later wrote a note of thanks to the researcher (Walker, 1989).

Informants are not always aware of their rights to refuse participation in the research, particularly if it lasts over a long period of time, and when unexpected elements arise. The researcher must understand the feeling of obligation that participants might have. Often they feel powerless to deny the researchers access to their world.

Platt (1981) states that in interview situations informants are often in a position of inequality. Colleagues and other health workers have more choice in accepting or rejecting participation because they are generally in a situation of power equal or similar to that of the researcher. When researchers interview and observe their peers, a more reciprocal relationship exists which makes it easier for participants to become equal partners in the research enterprise – the aim, of course, of most qualitative research. 'Researching one's peers' may mean, however, that researchers sometimes impose a framework which is based on the assumption of shared perceptions and does not allow informants to develop their own ideas.

Anonymity and confidentiality

Qualitative health care research might be more intrusive than quantitative research; therefore, the researcher needs sensitivity and communication skills. Usually, anonymity is guaranteed, and a promise is given that identities will not be revealed. Qualitative researchers work with small samples, and it is not always easy to protect identities. Even a detailed job description or an unusual occupational title of an informant may destroy anonymity. *Thick description* (Geertz, 1973), one of the characteristics of this type of research, means that everything is described in great detail, which might uncover the identity of the informant; this is why researchers must take care in the process

---

Example

The research of one of our students involved just one man, all other participants were women. She did not mention anything which could have identified him. Fortunately no gender issues arose which would have been important for the study, because the student could not have discussed these without disclosing the identity of the participant (Mayo, 1993).

Researchers sometimes change minor details so that informants cannot be recognised. For instance, researchers may change the age of all participants by 2 or 3 years when age is not an important factor in the research (Archbold, 1986).

Only the researcher should be able to match the real names and identities with the tapes, reports or descriptions, and participants are given pseudonyms. Tapes, notes and transcriptions – important tools for the qualitative researcher – are kept secure, and names should not be located near the tapes. If other people (superiors, supervisors or typists) have access to the information, however limited this might be, names should not be disclosed, participants' identities must be disguised, and they should be asked for permission.

The researcher's dilemma is to decide what information can be made public; if there is doubt or ambiguity, the decision depends upon the client's wishes. Some informants may allow details to be given about them which would identify them to some people, but this can create problems for the researcher; discussing these issues with the informants can therefore be useful.

Confidentiality is a separate issue from anonymity but also very important. In research where words and ideas from participants are used, full confidentiality cannot be promised. In these studies, confidentiality means that they keep that confidential which the participant does not wish to disclose to others. Patients, in particular, sometimes disclose intimate details of their lives which the researcher cannot divulge, although the information could be useful for the research.

To ensure anonymity, tapes of interviews should not carry names of informants but numbers or pseudonyms. The matching list of names is stored separately from the tapes. Videotapes, too, must be kept safe as participants are recognisable. It is suggested (Patton, 1990) that tapes should be erased a year after the research has been finished, but some ethics committees demand that they be kept for 10 years. We erased our tapes soon after the research was finished because that was the wish of the participants.

The dual role

Fowler (1988) focuses on role conflict in qualitative research. Nurses and midwives have a dual role and responsibility, that of professional and that of researcher, and they may experience problems of identity. On the one hand, they are committed to the research as they wish to advance health knowledge for the good of their clients and recognise that nursing and midwifery can only be professions if they become research-based. On the other hand, nurses and midwives are dedicated to the care and welfare of clients. Health professionals cannot close their eyes to distress and pain because their professional training guides them towards being carers and advocates for their clients. Fowler stresses that nurses have a duty to their patients first, as the profession mainly exists for its clients. If informants are threatened by the research or feel that they are, then the professional has to give up the researcher role.

Nurses and midwives must be clear not only about their own identity but about that of the client, which may pose a dilemma. In the professional role, they recognise the person as patient or client, while in their researcher role they see the person as an informant, as a participant in the research. The different elements of the professional identity cannot always be reconciled. Clients, too, do not always understand this duality and dichotomy in the health worker's role. They expect care and help from the person whom they perceive as a nurse or midwife and who professes to be a researcher.

Smith (1992) and Wilde (1992) stress the researcher's role as one of investigation rather than one of counselling or educating. Adopting the counselling or therapeutic role might shift the power balance and destroy the essential character of qualitative research, which is based on equality between researcher and informant. Clients must recognise that professional intervention by the researcher is not always possible. Nevertheless, health professionals cannot completely detach themselves from their informants, particularly in the close relationship of the qualitative research process. They respond to distress and need, especially in emergency situations, or call on colleagues who perform caring roles in the setting.

Example

One of our students, an experienced nurse who worked on a renal dialysis unit, interviewed a number of individuals about kidney transplant failures which had happened in the preceding year. Although the participants welcomed the interviews as they wanted to share their experiences, they also occasionally became distressed as the failure was an emotional event for them. Our student recognised this and followed the first principle of ethical research, never to leave a participant in distress (Mayo, 1993).

If nurses find strong distress, there is need for a mechanism for following up the participants. Perhaps a form of counselling could be built into the study. Robinson & Thorne (1988) state that the rights of the informants are more important than the interests of the researcher. Any interventions, however, should be made explicit in the research report.

Qualitative researchers must consider additional issues which are somewhat different from those of quantitative research. Power relationships might affect the research.

Example

Seibold *et al.* (1994) recount research experiences which Seibold had when interviewing a group of women in midlife. She found that the participants revealed parts of their lives which were highly personal. The women them-selves were surprised about these revelations, and the researcher had to be very sensitive about the interviews. This demonstrates, that consent given before the interview cannot be taken for granted and must be confirmed afterwards without putting pressure on the participants.

Mander (1988) claims that patients are particularly vulnerable because they are a captive population. While official documents focus on the rights of patients, research in nursing and midwifery often deals with people who have little real power in their situation. The power balance is perhaps more equal in the client's own setting than in the hospital situation.

Patients and clients rarely refuse when asked to take part in research as they feel dependent on the good will of carers. Because of the power differential, Archbold (1986) suggests that health professionals do not do research with people directly in their care. Occasionally, however, this cannot be avoided as the research might have been generated by a problem in the professional's own setting. Students do not always have access to settings other than their own.

Patients, of course, are vulnerable. Children, people with learning difficulties and those who have a mental or terminal illness need particular protection. Researchers are obliged to ask the parents or legal guardians for permission to research, not only the participants. Research should only be undertaken with these groups by experienced health professionals after careful consideration.

Empathy and research-mindedness

A research study requires both empathy and distancing. These traits appear con-tradictory. On the one hand, the researchers are asked to be non-judgmental and must be aware of personal values which could influence the research. On the other hand, health carers often have empathy and feelings for their clients. However involved, the researcher cannot allow preconceived attitudes or over-involvement to influence the data. This can be problematic because of the close relationship between the researcher and the participants (this is discussed elsewhere, e.g. in Chapter 9).

Researchers must be able to put themselves into the informant's place; this helps to establish rapport which is important in this type of approach. The researcher might therefore experience intense emotions. Qualitative research into sensitive topics generates these problems to a greater extent than any other type. Perhaps support for researchers is needed, for example they could co-counsel each other when doing this sort of research.

Interviews, in particular, may deeply affect participants who do not just reveal their experiences and thoughts to the researcher but sometimes become aware of hidden feelings themselves for the first time. The interview, in this case, can change the life of the informant, although the initial aim of the researcher is the collection of data which may or may not bring about change in the setting (Patton, 1990).

Towards the end of the research project another problem arises: the continuous, intimate nature of the interviewer–informant relationship generates trust and sometimes friendship; therefore, it is difficult for both researcher and participant to extricate themselves from it. A sensitive researcher does not leave the patient anxious or worried. May (1991) suggests the 'debriefing' of informants and the provision of emotional support if this is needed. This can be important for the interviewer, who might find these conversations distressing and stressful.

Research interviews can, of course, be therapeutic, although therapy is not the purpose of the interview. Lofland & Lofland (1984) suggest that there is often a *quid pro quo* in research. The researcher gains knowledge from informants who, in turn, find patient listeners for their feelings and thoughts. This means that reciprocity exists. Walker (1989), in her study on pain, relates that patients welcomed an opportunity to talk and found it beneficial.

Ethical questions arise in observation, too. Covert observation is problematic and its ethics debatable. Sapsford & Abbot (1992) suggest that in this type of research participants are sometimes deceived and exploited. Researchers in the field of health care generally disclose their presence as observers and reveal the purpose of the observation. However, this may generate the observer effect – the change that observers may bring about in the setting through their presence. Patton (1990) suggests that the effect is overestimated, as participants often forget the presence of the researcher. In any case, clients and colleagues generally trust the health professional to behave ethically.

Sometimes, however, non-disclosure of certain facts minimises the researcher effect.

Example

A ward sister wanted to explore bedside handover on her own ward from the patients' point of view. She explained this to her colleagues.

She intended to interview patients who had experienced several handovers, but felt that disclosure of her position in authority would bias the research. Patients might not be comfortable talking to a ward sister about matters that involved her colleagues and might feel obliged to give positive comments only.

Much debate about ethical issues took place between the researcher, her colleagues and her supervisor. In the end she asked patients' permission for interviews in her role as nurse researcher but did not disclose her ward sister role until the completion of individual interviews and gave patients the opportunity to opt out of the research. She did not lie about her position and would have disclosed it had she been asked. The researcher felt that in this way she did not compromise the veracity of the research which would then be accurate and truthful (Waltho, 1992).

Not everybody agreed with the solution to the problem, but difficult decisions must often be made by a researcher after balancing advantages and disadvantages of certain procedures. This form of initial deception is only justifiable because it produces accurate data without harming the informants. Sieber (1992:64,65) states: 'If it is to be acceptable at all, deception should not involve people in ways that members of the subject population would find unacceptable'. In the above example, all informants remained in the research.

Summary

Qualitative research generates difficult ethical questions. Apart from seeking access to the setting from gatekeepers and ethics committees, the researchers also, and most importantly, must ask permission from participants. The principles of ethical conduct must be followed and the rights and wishes of individuals taken into account in the research, particularly the right to make their own decisions. Anonymity and confidentiality must be respected. Participation can only be voluntary and the informants should be able to withdraw from the research, if they so wish, at any time.

The nurse or midwife researcher has conflicting roles, that of health professional and that of researcher. The search for rich and deep data may cause distress but informants should not be left worried or anxious because of their participation in the research.

It can be seen that nurses and midwives who attempt qualitative projects in clinical settings have to construct a complex ethical framework for the research, which is all the more important when dealing with patients and clients.

Acknowledgement

This chapter was published in an abridged version in: Holloway I.M. & Wheeler S.J. (1995) Ethics in qualitative research. *Nursing Ethics*, **2**, 223–232, published by Edward Arnold, London.

References

Archbold P. (1986) Ethical issues in qualitative research. In *From Practice to Grounded Theory: Qualitative Research in Nursing* (eds W.C. Cheritz & J.M. Swanson), pp. 155–163, Addison-Wesley, Menlo Park, California.

Beauchamp T.L. & Childress J.F. (1994) *Principles of Biomedical Ethics* 4th edn. Oxford University Press, New York.

Clarke J. (1991) Moral dilemmas in nursing research. *Nursing Practice*, **4**, 22–25.

Couchman W. & Dawson J. (1995) *Nursing and Health-Care Research* 2nd edn. Scutari Press, London.

Cowles K.V. (1988) Issues in qualitative research on sensitive topics. *Western Journal of Nursing Research*, **10**(2), 163–179.

Ford J.S. & Reutter L.I. (1990) Ethical dilemmas associated with small samples. *Journal of Advanced Nursing*, **15**, 187–191.

Fowler M.D.M. (1988) Ethical issues in nursing research, **10**, 109–111.

Geertz C. (1973) *The Interpretation of Cultures*. Basic Books, New York.

Lofland J. & Lofland L. (1984) *Analysing Social Settings* 2nd edn. Wadsworth, Belmont, California.

Mander R. (1988) Encouraging students to be research minded. *Nurse Education Today*, **8**, 30–35.

May K.A. (1991) Interview techniques in qualitative research: concerns and challenges. In *Qualitative Nursing Research: A Contemporary Dialogue* (ed. J.M. Morse) pp. 188–201, Sage, London.

Mayo A. (1993) The meaning of transplant failure. Unpublished BSc project, Bournemouth University, Bournemouth.

Patton M.Q. (1990) *Qualitative Evaluation and Research Methods* 2nd edn. Sage, London.

Platt J. (1981) On interviewing one's peers. *British Journal of Sociology*, **32**(1), 75–91.

Robinson C.A. & Thorne S.E. (1988) Dilemmas of ethics and validity in qualitative nursing research. *The Canadian Journal of Nursing Research*, **20**, 65–76.

Sapsford R. & Abbot P. (1992) *Research Methods for Nurses and the Caring Professions*. Open University Press, Milton Keynes.

Seibold C., Richards L. & Simon D. (1994) Feminist method and qualitative research about midlife. *Journal of Advanced Nursing*, **19**, 394–402.

Sieber J.E. (1992) *Planning Ethically Responsible Research*. Sage, London.

Sim J. (1991) Nursing research: is there an obligation to participate? *Journal of Advanced Nursing*, **16**, 1284–1289.

Smith L. (1992) Ethical issues in interviewing. *Journal of Advanced Nursing*, **17**, 98–103.

Tschudin V. (1986) *Ethics in Nursing: The Caring Relationship*. Heinemann Nursing, London.

Tschudin V. (1992) *Ethics in Nursing: The Caring Relationship* 2nd edn. Butterworth Heinemann, Oxford.

United Kingdom Central Council for Nursing, Midwifery and Health Visiting (1992) *Code of Professional Conduct* 3rd edn. UKCC, London.

Walker J. (1989) The management of elderly patients with pain: a community nursing perspective. Unpublished PhD thesis, Bournemouth University, Bournemouth.

Waltho B.J. (1992) Perception of the nurse–patient relationship: patients' perceptions of bedside handover. BSc project, Bournemouth Polytechnic (now University), Bournemouth.

Wilde V. (1992) Controversial hypotheses on the relationship between researcher and informant in qualitative research. *Journal of Advanced Nursing*, **17**, 234–242.

World Medical Association (1964, revised 1975) *The Declaration of Helsinki*.

Chapter 4

Data Collection in Qualitative Research

In this chapter we shall describe:

- The interviewing process
- Narratives and life histories
- Participant observation
- Documentary sources
- Practical considerations

The description of data collection is important, because without it the reader cannot understand the research process adequately. Researchers collect their data through interviewing, observing or through documentary search once they have decided on a research question; sometimes they even use films, photographs or videotapes. In this chapter the process of data collection will be described.

The interviewing process

The most common form of data gathering is interviewing. Health professionals are used to interviewing people. In their everyday work they have conversations with their clients to gain information from them. Nurses might assume therefore that research interviews are easy, but they are not as simple as they seem. Many researchers have found that patients often give monosyllabic answers until they have become used to the interviewer, because they see the interview as an assessment of their condition.

Burgess (1984) maintains that qualitative interviews are 'conversations with a purpose' and shows that many of the initial research interviews consist of informal questions and answers. The research interview is more than a conversation and ranges from the informal to the formal. Although all conversations have certain rules of turntaking or control by one or other of the participants, the rules of research interviews are stricter. Unlike some conversations, they are set up to elicit information from one side only, therefore an asymmetrical relationship exists (Spradley, 1979), however much the interviewer attempts to achieve a relationship of equality with the participant. The researchers tend to guide interviews towards the discovery of informants' feelings, perceptions and thoughts.

In our experience students become more confident as interviews proceed. May (1991) tells us that the interview can be formal, that is, pre-planned for the express purpose of eliciting information, but often chance meetings and informal conversations with participants generate important ideas for the project. Although pilot studies are not usual in qualitative enquiry, novice researchers could try interviews with their friends and acquaintances to get used to this type of data collection. We found that we lacked confidence when we started, and a practice run proved very useful.

One-to-one interviews are the most common form of data collection. Examples can be given from much nursing research; for instance Melia (1987) interviewed student nurses about learning their roles in the clinical setting. She acquired her knowledge by talking to individuals.

Sometimes researchers use focus group interviews, that is, they interview a group of people who have shared the experience of an illness or a professional specialism, for instance a group of patients with diabetes or a group of paediatric nurses. Occasionally, a number of interviewers are involved in interviewing a variety of participants. A good example is the now classic and famous study by Becker *et al.* (1961) in which the writers examined the process of socialisation into the profession of medicine and illustrated how young doctors learn their professional roles. Becker and his co-researchers not only observed them in the hospital setting but also interviewed them about their behaviour. As the study was large and complex, several interviewers and observers were needed.

In student projects, dissertations and theses, however, the one-to-one interview is prevalent, either in a single encounter or in several meetings with individual participants. In qualitative enquiry it is possible to re-examine the issues in the light of emerging ideas and interview for a second or third time. Seidmann (1991) sees three interviews as the optimum number, but this would be difficult in the short time span available to undergraduates for their project. Many qualitative researchers use one interview.

Most qualitative research starts with relatively unstructured interviews in which researchers give minimal guidance to the participants. The outcome of initial interviews guides later stages of interviewing. As interviews proceed, they become more focused on the particular issues which are important to the participants and emerge throughout the data collection. Flexibility and consistency must be balanced in the research (May, 1991) so that health professionals can compare the accounts of individuals without neglecting the unique stories of their experience.

Types of interview

Researchers have to decide on the amount of structure in the interview. One can trace a continuum of interview types, from the unstructured to the structured interview. Qualitative researchers generally employ the unstructured or semi-structured interview.

The unstructured, non-standardised interview

Unstructured interviews start with a general question in the broad area of study. Even unstructured interviews are usually accompanied by an *aide mémoire*, an agenda or a list of topics which will be covered in the interviews. There are, however, no predetermined questions except in the very beginning of the interview.

Example

Tell me about your experience of pain.

Aide mémoire
Feelings
Visits to doctor
Other professionals
Use of complementary medicine
Social support
Practical support
Pain clinic
Peaks of pain

This type of unstructured interviewing allows flexibility and makes it possible for researchers to follow the interests and thoughts of the informants. Interviewers freely ask questions from informants in any order or sequence depending on the answers. These are followed up, but researchers also have their own agenda: the research aim they have in mind and the particular issues which they wish to explore. However, direction and control of the interview by the researcher is minimal. Generally, the outcomes of these interviews differ for each informant, though usually certain patterns can be discerned. Informants are free to answer at length, and great depth and detail can be obtained.

Patton (1990) suggests that this kind of interview is particularly appropriate when the researcher interviews the participant more than once. The unstructured interview generates the richest data, but it also has the highest 'dross rate' (the amount of material of no particular use for the researcher's study), particularly with an inexperienced interviewer.

The semi-structured interview

Semi-structured or focused interviews are often used in qualitative research. The questions are contained in an interview guide (not a schedule as in quantitative research) with a focus on the issues to be covered. The sequencing of questions is not the same for every participant as it depends on the process of the interview and the answers of each individual. The interview guide, however, ensures that the researcher collects similar types of data from all informants. In this way, the interviewer can save time. The dross rate is lower than in unstructured interviews. Researchers can develop questions and decide for themselves which issues to pursue.

> **Example**
>
> Tell me how your pain first started?
> Did you go and tell the doctor at any stage in the early days?
> What did he/she say?
> What happened after that?
>   and so on . . .

The interview guide can be quite long and detailed although it need not be followed strictly. Burgess (1984) suggests that the longer the questions, the longer the answers. We have had quite different experiences when talking to our students or other nurse researchers and find good questions of medium length with the use of prompts more useful. The interview guide focuses on particular aspects of the subject area to be examined, but it can be revised after interviewing because of the ideas that arise. Although interviewers aim to gain the informants' perspectives, they must remember that they need some control of the interview so that the purpose of the study can be achieved and the research topic explored. Ultimately, the researchers themselves must decide what interview techniques might be best for them and the interview participants.

The structured or standardised interview

Qualitative researchers rarely use standardised interviews. The interview schedule contains a number of pre-planned questions. Each informant is asked the same questions in the same order. This type of interview resembles a written survey questionnaire. Standardised interviews save time and limit the interviewer effect when a number of different interviewers are involved in the research. The analysis of the data seems easier as answers can be found quickly. Generally, knowledge of statistics is important and useful for the analysis of this type of interview. However, this type of pre-planned interview directs the informants' responses and is therefore inappropriate in qualitative approaches. Structured interviews may contain open questions, but researchers must be warned against these as methodological issues get muddled and the analysis will be difficult.

Qualitative researchers use structured questions only to elicit socio-demographic data, i.e. about age, length of condition, length of experience, type of occupation, qualifications, etc. Sometimes research or ethics committees ask for a pre-determined interview schedule so that they can find out the exact path of the research. In this case, a semi-structured interview guide would be advisable for nursing researchers.

Length and timing of interviews

Field & Morse (1985) advise that interviews should not be continued beyond 1 hour. We feel that the length of time depends on the informant. Of course, the researcher must suggest an approximate amount of time so that participants can plan their day , but many are willing or wish to go beyond this. Others, particularly elderly people or physically weak informants, might need to break off after a short while, say 20 or 30 minutes. Children cannot concentrate for long periods of time. Nurses and midwives have to use their own judgment, follow the wishes of the informant and take the length of time required for the topic. One of our colleagues suggests that 3 hours should be the absolute maximum because concentration fails even an experienced researcher.

The statement of an approximate time for the interview before its start can ensure escape for the researcher when participants wish to tell them their whole life history. For hard-pressed nurses these types of interview are very time-consuming, however useful and therapeutic they may be for for the informant. As stated before, researchers can, of course, re-interview one or more times – Field & Morse (1985:67) suggest that 'several short interviews are more effective than one long one'.

Types of questions

When asking questions, interviewers use a variety of techniques. Patton (1990) lists particular types of questions, for example experience, feeling and knowledge questions.

Examples

Experience question:
Could you tell me about your experience of caring for patients with diabetes?

Feeling question:
How did you feel when the first patient in your care died?

Knowledge question:
What services are available for this group of patients?

Spradley (1979) distinguishes between grand tour and mini-tour questions. Grand tour questions are broader, while mini-tour questions are more specific.

Examples

Grand tour questions:
Can you describe a typical day on the ward?
What do you do when patients ask you about their condition?

Mini-tour question:
Can you describe what happens when a colleague questions your decision?

In qualitative studies questions are as non-directive as possible but still guide towards the area of study which is of interest to the researcher. Researchers phrase questions clearly and aim at the participants' level of understanding. Ambiguous questions lead to ambiguous answers. Double questions are best avoided; for instance it would be inappropriate to ask: How many colleagues do you have, and what are their ideas about this?

Probing and prompting

During the interviews researchers can use prompts or probing questions. These help to reduce both researcher and research informant anxiety. The purpose of probes is a search for elaboration, meaning or reasons. Seidman (1991) prefers the term *explore* and dislikes the word *probe* as it stresses the interviewer's position of power and is the name for an instrument used in medical or dental investigations. Exploratory questions might be, for instance: What was that experience like for you? How did you feel about that? Can you tell me more about that? That's interesting, why did you do that?

Non-verbal prompts are perhaps even more useful. The stance of the researcher, eye contact and leaning forwards encourage reflection. In fact, some of the listening skills adopted in counselling which some nurses already possess will elicit further ideas.

The interviewer can follow up certain points that participants make or words they use. They become fluent talkers when asked to tell a story, reconstructing their experiences, for instance a day, an incident or the feeling about an illness.

Interviewing colleagues

Many health professionals have an interest in the views and ideas of their colleagues. There are advantages and disadvantages in interviewing one's peers. Shared language and norms can be advantageous or problematic. Concepts are more easily understood by a researcher who is involved in the culture of the participants. Although there is less room for misinterpretation, misunderstandings can arise from the assumptions of common values and beliefs. Thoughts that are uncovered or constructs which arise might not be questioned. The researcher can overcome this by acting as *cultural stranger* or *naive* observer, asking participants about their meaning and for clarification of their ideas.

In many interview situations with peers, researcher and informant are in a position of equality (Platt, 1981) and the researcher is not distant or anonymous. This has advantages in that the participants will 'open up' and trust researchers, but there is the danger of over-involvement and identification with participants. In some cases it may be possible for the researcher to overcome this involvement with peers and elicit responses from research informants outside the shared frame of reference (Hudson, 1986).

> Example
>
> S.W. investigated health visitors' and social workers' perceptions of child abuse. She was anxious to avoid over-identification with the members of her own profession, health visiting, with whom she shared the frame of reference. This, she thought, might prejudice the information. As part of the background to her study, she visited Dr Dingwall at Wolfson College, Oxford, who had done academic work in the field of child abuse. He suggested interviewing the social workers first and using some of the information from the transcripts to interview the health visitors. She then presented the perceptions of the social workers to the health visitors for comment. There was a shift of focus so that her own background did not interfere (Wheeler, 1989).

Students, however, sometimes interview friends and acquaintances for pragmatic and opportunistic reasons. Although this is useful in order to overcome the hurdles of getting to know informants and forming relationships, the selection from this group might create unease or embarrassment if the topic is a sensitive one. Informants and interviewers might hold assumptions about each other which might prejudice the information. Therefore we suggest that students take great care in their choice of informants.

Narratives and life histories

Narratives and life histories are stories which individuals tell about their condition, work or life. They are not new forms of data collection but have existed for centuries as autobiographies, diaries, oral histories or travellers' tales. In the past, narratives were not analysed systematically nor did they always form part of a research approach. They have found a place in naturalistic enquiry because they are in tune with the world view of qualitative researchers. Narratives are especially useful for studying 'the phenomena of development and transition in people's lives' (Josselson & Lieblich, 1993:ix). Researchers analyse and search for meaning so that the story is transformed from a journalistic report or literary text into academic research. They must realise, however, that narratives are already interpretations or modifications of reality, not merely a factual account of events.

Authors can focus on single cases – looking at the story of one individual – or multiple case studies through which they explore the lives of a group of people. Narratives as data are most often collected by nurses and midwives who have an interest in the psychological factors which affect people.

There is only a slight difference between these methods and unstructured interviews: narratives are 'long stretches of talk' (Riessman, 1993). The interviewer asks very few questions and encourages the participants to tell their own story. The use of narratives is intended to focus on people's accounts of their own lives

(Marshall & Rossman, 1995). They reconstruct their stories and relive their experiences.

> ## Example
>
> Kleinman (1988), the psychiatrist and anthropologist, collected the illness narratives of his patients. They are full of the deep feelings of suffering and pain which individuals experience when they are ill. These narratives are the stories of people with chronic illness who talk of their pain and vulnerability.

Through narratives and life histories, nurses can identify people's feelings, beliefs and actions, but only if they are thoughtful and sensitive listeners. Researchers learn how events from the past have influenced patients or colleagues.

Riessman (1993) distinguishes between three types of narrative. First, in habitual narratives, routine events and actions are recalled. An example would be a day on a ward or in the life of a district nurse. Second, hypothetical narratives describe events which did not take place. An imaginary story would be an example of this. Third, topic-centred narratives are stories of past events which are connected thematically by the story-teller. The report of the progress of an illness would be a topic-centred narrative.

> ## Example
>
> Robinson (1990) asked people with multiple sclerosis to write stories about life events and feelings which they experienced. The study showed that these individuals tried to make sense of their condition and wanted to achieve mastery over it.

It must be remembered that narratives are interpretations; while telling the story people give meaning to that which happened to them. These stories are given in simple natural language. The participants generally recall most vividly the events and actions which have influenced them or made a strong impression. Riessman (1993) shows that the person who has an experience tells a tale to the listener who was not there when it happened. The story-tellers want to recreate feelings which they had and transmit them to other people.

The narrative is a powerful means through which researchers and readers can gain access to the world of participants and share their experiences. Patients who live with an illness and experience pain can assist researchers who wish to learn about people's own perceptions.

> ### Example
>
> Viney & Bousfield (1991) interviewed people suffering from AIDS who showed strong emotions when talking about their condition. The researchers demonstrated that narratives mirror the meanings and experiences of people more closely than other methods because the sufferers are allowed to tell the story in their own way.

Viney & Bousfield (1991) believe that telling stories can empower people and help them to order their experiences. Examples of questions which encourage participants to report on their lives are, for instance: Tell me what happened, or tell me about your feelings and thoughts at that time. As in unstructured interviewing, open-ended questions are the most appropriate. The collection of these life histories is a lengthy process which can go on over several months of weekly meetings.

Life histories differ from narratives by being structured in a chronological sequence which covers a long period of time. They are individuals' perspectives on their own lives and development, sometimes including work or illness careers. The nurse can use them in research with patients or colleagues. Hagemaster (1992) asserts that this method of data collection allows researchers to identify health patterns or health beliefs of patients, and they can be useful in demonstrating how early experiences influence later events.

> ### Example
>
> A counsellor who worked with alcoholic women wanted to know about the lived experience of these individuals. She planned a series of interviews with them to explore the culture of excessive alcohol consumption. Through non-judgmental questions, and an examination of the whole life history of these people, the counsellor gained a picture of the ways in which individuals became addicted and some of the reasons for this.

Life histories help nurses to understand not only the personal lives of patients or colleagues, they might also learn about a culture and its values and norms. More importantly, nurses might come to understand the reasons for people's beliefs and behaviour.

Participant observation

Another strategy for the collection of data is observation. When researchers become observers, they do not set up artificial situations but look at places and people in their natural settings. For nurse and midwifery observers this may be a ward, a reception area, a clinic or any other relevant location inside the hospital or in the community. Qualitative researchers generally use participant observation, a term originally coined by Lindeman (in Bogdewic, 1992) which he described as the exploration of a culture from the inside. As Jorgenson (1989:15) states: 'Participant observation provides direct experiential and observational access to the insiders' world of meaning'. The social reality of the people observed is examined.

Participant observation has its origins in anthropology and sociology. As stated before, from the early days of fieldwork, anthropologists and sociologists became part of the culture they studied and examined the actions and interactions of people in their social context, 'in the field'. Famous studies in anthropology are those of Mead (1935) and Malinowski (1922) on other cultures. In sociology, the participant observations of Strauss and his colleagues in psychiatric hospitals (Strauss *et al.*, 1964) and Spradley's work with tramps in the 1960s (Spradley, 1970) typify some of the early, well-known studies. Immersion in a setting can take a long time, often many years of living in a culture. Participant observation in clinical settings too, goes on over some time, often over a year or years (Atkinson, 1981; Roth, 1963), although some observation does not take as long. It must be remembered that nurses and other health professionals are members of the culture they examine and know it well, therefore they may not need a long introduction; however, because of this they may miss important events or behaviours in the setting they study.

Prolonged observation generates more in-depth knowledge of a culture or subculture, and researchers can avoid disturbances and potential biases caused by an occasional visit from an unknown stranger. Observation is less disruptive and more unobtrusive than interviewing. However, participant observation does not just involve observing the situation, but also listening to the people under study.

The location

Nurse researchers can observe any appropriate setting which becomes the focus for their study. Participant observation varies on a continuum from open to closed settings. Open settings are public and highly visible, such as street scenes, hospital corridors and reception areas. In closed settings, access is difficult; doctors' surgeries, management meetings or clinics can be considered closed settings.

Types of observation

The participant observer enters the setting without intention to limit the observation to particular processes or people and adopts an unstructured approach. Occasionally certain foci crystallise early in the study, but usually observation progresses from the unstructured to the more focused until eventually specific actions and events become the main interest of the researcher.

Gold (1958) identified four types of observer involvement in the field.

(1)   The complete participant
(2)   The participant as observer
(3)   The observer as participant
(4)   The complete observer

The complete participant

The complete participant is part of the setting and takes an insider role which involves covert observation.

Examples

Roth (1963), an American sociologist, was a patient in a tuberculosis hospital. While being part of the setting, he observed the interaction of patients with the health personnel, focusing on negotiation concerning time spent in and out of hospital.

The best known study of covert observation is that of Rosenhan (1973) who wanted to discover whether 'sane' and 'insane' individuals could be distinguished by health professionals. Eight pseudo patients were sent to psychiatric hospitals where they exhibited 'normal' behaviour apart from an initial statement that they could hear voices. (All except one were labelled schizophrenic, with schizophrenia in remission, by health professionals, while other patients recognised their sanity.)

Rosenhan (1973) wished to show that notions of normality and abnormality are not as clear and unambiguous as is sometimes believed.

In spite of the value of this study, complete participation generates a number of problems. First of all, one would have to question seriously whether covert observation in care settings, without knowledge or permission of the people observed, is ethical. After all, this is not a public, open situation such as a street corner or rally, where nobody can be identified. For health professionals who advocate caring and ethical behaviour, covert observation would be inadvisable.

The participant as observer

Participants as observers have negotiated their way into the setting, and as observers they are part of the work group under study. For nursing researchers this seems a good way of doing research as they are already involved in the work situation. Many nurses and midwives wish to examine a problem in their ward or in the hospital. They ask permission from the relevant gatekeepers and participants and explain their observer roles to them. The first advantage of this type of observation is the ease with which researcher–participant relationships can be forged or extended. Secondly, the observers can move around in the location as they wish, and thus observe in more detail and depth.

For new researchers, observation is more difficult than interviewing because of the ethical issues involved. Patients have to be protected from intrusion when interaction with health professionals is explored. To ask all patients in a particular ward to give permission to participate, though difficult, may be possible, but ethics committees are often reluctant to allow young students to observe. It is easier for experienced nurses or midwives to gain access.

The observer as participant

These observers are only marginally involved in the situation. For instance, nurses might observe a ward but do not directly work as part of the work force; they have, however, announced their interest and their public role and gone through the process of gaining entry. The advantage of this type of observation is the possibility for the nurse to ask questions and be accepted as a colleague and researcher, but not called upon as a member of the work force. On the other hand, observers are prevented from playing a real role in the setting, and this restraint from involvement is not easy, particularly in a busy work situation. Researchers must always ask permission from those in the setting.

The complete observer

Complete observers do not take part in the setting and use a 'fly on the wall' approach. Observations in reception areas or in an accident and emergency department are examples of this. The complete observer situation is really only possible when the researcher observes through a two-way mirror in a public setting where he or she is not noticed and has no impact on the situation. This is commonly used in child guidance clinics in order to observe family interaction. Again, permission from participants should be sought.

Three step progression

Spradley (1980) claims that observers progress in three steps; they use descriptive, focused and finally selective observation. Descriptive observation proceeds on the basis of general questions that the observer has in mind. Everything that goes on in the situation becomes data and is recorded, including colours, smells and appearances of people in the setting. Description involves all five senses. As time goes by, certain important areas or aspects of the setting become more obvious and the researcher focuses on these because they contribute to the achievement of the aim of the research. Eventually the observation becomes highly selective.

LeCompte & Preissle (1993) give guidelines for observations which we will summarise.

(1) *The 'who' questions.* How many people are present in the setting or take part in the activities? What are their characteristics and roles?

(2) *The 'what' questions.* What is happening in the setting? What are the actions and rules of behaviour? What are the variations in the behaviour observed?

(3) *The 'where' questions.* Where do interactions take place? Where are people located in the physical space?

(4) *The 'when' questions.* When do conversations and interactions take place? What is the timing of activities?

(5) The 'why' questions. Why do people in the setting act the way they do? Why are there variations in behaviour?

Mini-tour observation leads to detailed descriptions of smaller settings, while grand-tour observations are more appropriate for larger settings. After the initial stages, certain dimensions and features of observation become interesting to the researcher, who then proceeds to observe these dimensions specifically. 'Progressive focusing' (discussed earlier) is not just a feature of interviewing but also of observation.

Example

A nurse who has previously observed interactions and events on the ward, notices that at certain times patients tend to grow restless. She or he becomes interested in this phenomenon and tries to discover the reasons for this restlessness.

If the nurse observed more specific ways of interacting in particular situations, the study becomes more focused. Focused observations are the outcome of specific questions. From broader observations researchers proceed to observing small units which they want to investigate. This may be a handover on the ward or an assessment. The researchers look for similarities and differences among groups and individuals. For this type of observation a narrow focus and specificity are useful and necessary.

Marshall and Rossman (1995:79) state that 'observation entails the systematic noting and recording of events, behaviours and artifacts (objects) in the social setting chosen for study'. The situation can then be analysed. Nurses and midwives observe social processes as they happen and develop. The observers can examine events and ongoing actions, they cannot explore past events and thoughts of participants. This is only possible in interviews. Usually though, interviewing is seen as part of participant observation. The study by Becker and his colleagues (1961) shows this clearly: the participants, medical students, were observed in their interaction with patients, colleagues and teachers, and the researchers then asked questions about what they saw and heard. Hammersley & Atkinson (1995), in fact, propose that one might see all social research as participant observation to the extent that the researcher actively participates in the situation.

Nurses and other health professionals sometimes shy away from formal participant observation because of problems of access, ethics and time. For instance, it is easier to obtain permission to interview colleagues than to observe them, because any observation would include observing patients. Observation might change the situation, as people act differently when they are observed, although they often forget the presence of the observer in long-term observation. The latter, however, takes more time than is practical in student projects, although it is often used by post-graduates and experienced researchers.

When observations are successful, they can uncover interesting patterns and developments which have their basis in the real world of the daily life of the participants, and the task of exploration and discovery is, after all, the aim of qualitative research.

Documentary sources

The third type of data consists of written documents and records. Hammersley & Atkinson (1995) suggest that researchers use these because they give information about situations which cannot be investigated by direct observation or questioning. The documents are collected and analysed in both qualitative and quantitative research, but generally in the former. They consist typically of personal diaries, letters, autobiographies and biographies but also of official documents and reports; that is they range from informal documentary sources to formal and official reports such as newspapers or minutes of meetings. Timetables, case notes and reports can become the focus of nurses' investigation. The researcher treats them like transcriptions of interviews or detailed descriptions of observations, that is, they are coded and categorised. They act as sensitising devices and make researchers aware of important issues.

Example

Hawker (1991) examined the patterns of care in two Dorset parishes between the years 1700 and 1799. She investigated the records in the County Record Office to find out how medical care and nursing care were administered to sick poor people in two parishes. As there were few diaries and letters she looked at the overseer reports and accounts (an overseer of the poor was appointed by the parishes), and from this she gleaned which people helped the poor and how they did so.

Many of these texts exist before researchers start their work, others are initiated and organised by the researchers themselves. Historical documents, archives and products of the media exist independently from researchers, while personal diaries might be written through their intervention or instigation; for instance Hammersley & Atkinson (1995) cite a study of a midwife who used personal diaries in her research on student midwives.

Scott (1990) differentiates between types of document by referring to them as closed, restricted and open-archival and open-published. Access to closed documents is limited to a few people, namely their authors and those who commissioned them. As far as restricted documents are concerned, researchers can only gain access with the permission of insiders under particular conditions.

Example

Nettleton & Harding (1994) examined all informal letters of complaint to a Family Health Service Authority in 1990. They analysed those complaints which did not proceed to a hearing. (These letters showed that patients, their relatives and friends complained about practitioners' non-responses to requests, their personal behaviour, and the health professionals' perceived mistakes.)

Permission for access is asked from the living authors of diaries and keepers of other confidential documents. Open-archival documents are available to any person, subject to administrative conditions and opening hours of libraries. Published documents, of course, can be accessed by anybody at any time.

Qualitative researchers most often seek access to diaries – which are people's own accounts of their lives – and letters, but also to historical documents or the products of the media. Merriam (1988) stresses the non-reactivity of documentary data and claims that they are grounded in their context which makes them useful and rich sources of information for researchers. Some researchers encourage participants to keep a diary for analysis. For instance, Seibold *et al.* (1994) relate that one of the researchers on whose research they report, encouraged the participants to keep a diary for 12 months.

Through documents researchers in the health professions acquire a perspective on history which gives them insiders' views on past lives and attitudes, or they can analyse contemporary documents, such as articles and comments in the press, and become aware of the significant features of issues or the dramatisation of particular events. Last, and most importantly, health professionals can trace the perspectives of diary or autobiography writers by collecting, reading and analysing these personal documents. Through this researchers can gain knowledge of the experiences of others in a particular context and at a particular time.

Researchers must be concerned about four major criteria which determine the quality of the documents: authenticity, credibility, representativeness and meaning (Scott, 1990). To demonstrate authenticity for historical documents, questions about their history as well as their writers' intentions and biases must be asked. Credibility too, involves some of these questions. Accuracy might be affected by the writers' proximity in time and place to the events described and also the conditions under which the information was acquired at the time. Representativeness of documents is difficult to prove because researchers often have no information of the numbers or variety of documents about a particular event.

Scott (1990) claims that the most significant aim of the collection and analysis of documents is the interpretation of their meanings. It is far easier to analyse a personal contemporary document, where the researcher is familiar with language and context, than to assess the representativeness or authenticity of a historical document whose context can only be assumed. Therefore, the researcher can only try to interpret the meaning of the text in context, study the situation and conditions in which it is written and try to establish the writer's intentions.

As in other types of data, the meaning is tentative and provisional only and may change when new data present a challenge and demand reappraisal. Hammersley & Atkinson (1995) warn that documents may generate biases as they are often written by and for élites or people in power. That in itself can be useful because not many sources exist that give the ideas of these informants.

As we have explained in Chapter 1, researchers sometimes triangulate within method. One such study is that of McClelland & Sands (1993), who collected their data through participant observation, interviewing and written and audio-visual record.

Practical considerations

A number of techniques and practical points must be considered so that the data are recorded and stored appropriately.

Interview data are recorded in three ways:

(1)   Tape-recording the interview
(2)   Note taking during the interview
(3)   Note taking after the interview

Tape-recording

Before analysing the data, researchers must preserve the words of the people they interview as accurately as possible. The best form of recording interview data is tape-recording. As we said before, nurses must ask for permission before taping informants' words. Because tapes contain the exact words of the interview, inclusive of questions, researchers do not make the mistake of forgetting important areas. The interviewer can have eye contact and pay attention to what participants say. Occasionally informants change their minds about tape-recording, and their wishes should be paramount for the researcher. The principle of respect for autonomy which concerns an individual's self-rule and choice, as previously stated, must be considered first in terms of consent. This allows for the right to refuse participation in research. This right can be exercised at any stage of the research process.

Initially the informants may be hesitant, but they will get used to the tape-recorder; a small recorder is easier to forget than a large one, but a larger recorder can be placed further away so it is not necessarily always visible to the participants. By asking factual questions first, researchers allow the informants to relax and make them feel more secure. Some interviewees have soft and quiet voices, particularly if they feel vulnerable. Interviewers therefore place the tape-recorder near enough, but not so prominently that it intimidates the hesitant person. A room away from noise and disturbances enhances not only the quality of the tape but also the interview itself as participants feel free to talk without interruption.

We have experienced some problems with tape recorders. They sometimes break down, and it is advisable to try them out at the beginning of the interview and after it has been recorded. When checking batteries before going to meet the informant, researchers should remember to pack some extra batteries. It is useful to bring extra tapes. A new recording device is available, a portable mini compact disc player which is, however, expensive. Each disc records 70 minutes and does not need to be turned over. Auto-reverse on tape-recorders is useful; standard cassettes need not be turned over and are longer (the quality of non-standard tape, for instance 90-minute tape, is not always very good). It is much better to use tape-recorders with conference facility, although we know that students often find them too expensive and have no access to them.

After the interviews the tape is dated and labelled. Pseudonyms only appear on the tape or its transcription, and participants' names and pseudonyms are stored in a different place from the tapes.

Transcription of tapes

The fullest and richest data can be gained from transcribing all interviews verbatim. We advise that, if possible, students transcribe their own tapes because this way they immerse themselves in the data. This process lasts a long time as 1 hour of interviewing takes between 4 and 6 hours of transcription. For those who are not used to audio-typing, it can be much longer. Transcribing is very frustrating and can take time which the researcher does not always have. It could be done more quickly by a typist using a transcribing machine, but it would be expensive. On the other hand, this would give more time to the researcher to listen and analyse. The decision about this depends on the researcher. Any outsider who transcribes must, of course, be advised on the confidentiality related to the data.

Initial interviews and field notes should be fully transcribed so that the researcher becomes aware of the important issues in the data. Novice researchers should transcribe all interviews, while more experienced individuals can be more selective in their transcriptions and transcribe that which is linked to their developing theoretical ideas. It is always better that the interviews or field notes are fully transcribed by the researchers themselves if they have the time. Pages are numbered, and the face sheet should contain date, location and time of interview, as well as the code number or letter for the informant. Many researchers number each line of the interview transcript so that they can find the data when searching for them.

A minimum of three copies (usually more) should be made of the transcripts, including a clean copy without comments for locking away in a safe place in case other copies are lost or destroyed.

Taking notes

Some researchers use the tape-recorder and take notes during the interview so that participants' facial expressions and gestures and interviewers' reactions and comments can be recorded. This method was used when one of us was interviewed last year (I.H.). The researcher tape-recorded the interview and wrote notes while keeping eye contact at the same time. This was very disturbing for the participant who wondered about the contents of the notes during the whole of the interview. We would suggest only to take notes during interviews when taping is not feasible or if interviewees do not wish to be tape-recorded.

However, when participants deny permission to be taped or when taping seems inappropriate, for instance in very sensitive situations, interviewers generally take notes throughout the interview, and these notes reflect the words of the participants as accurately as possible. As interviewers can only write down a fraction of the sentences, they select the most important words or phrases and summarise the rest. Patton (1990) advises on conventions in the use of quotation marks while writing notes. Researchers use them only for full, direct quotations from informants. He suggests that researchers adopt a mechanism for differentiating between one's own thoughts and informants' words.

Another way of recording is to take notes after the interview is finished. This should be done as soon as possible after the interview to capture the flavour, behaviour and words of the informants and the concomitant thoughts of the researcher. It should not be done in the presence of the participants.

The process of listening to the tapes will sensitise researchers to the data and uncover ambiguities or problems within them. At this time, any theoretical ideas that emerge should be written down in the form of memos (see Chapter 7).

Summary

Data are collected through unstructured or semi-structured interviews, participant observation and documents. The qualitative research interview is relatively non-directive and depends largely on the participants, whose ideas and thoughts researchers try to follow. The interview tends to become progressively focused as researchers develop sensitivity towards significant issues.

In participant observation, the researchers immerse themselves in the setting. They observe and describe it in detail, focusing mainly on interaction and other behaviours. Researchers also look at documents, be they diaries, letters or historical writing. Even videos, films or photographs can be part of the data collection. Audio-taping is the most common way of recording interviews; observations are sometimes video-taped, and occasionally, particularly during observation, researchers take notes. The recording of data depends on ethical and access considerations, that is, the permission of participants and gatekeepers.

References

Atkinson P.A. (1981) *The Clinical Experience*. Gower, Farnborough.

Becker H.S. *et al.* (1961) *Boys in White*. University of Chicago Press, New Brunswick.

Bogdewic S.P. (1992) Participant observation. In *Doing Qualitative Research* (eds B.F. Crabtree & W.L. Miller), pp. 45–269, Sage, Newbury Park, California.

Burgess R. G. (1984) *In the Field: An Introduction for Field Research*. Unwin Hyman, London.

Field P.A. & Morse J.M. (1985) *Nursing Research: The Application of Qualitative Approaches*. Croom Helm, London.

Gold R. (1958) Roles in sociological field observation. *Social Forces*, **36**, 217–223.

Hagemaster J.N. (1992) Life history: a qualitative method of research. *Journal of Advanced Nursing*, **17**, 1122–1128.

Hammersley M. & Atkinson P.A. (1995) *Ethnography: Principles in Practice* 2nd edn. Tavistock, London.

Hawker J. (1991) An investigation into patterns of care in two dorset parishes, 1700–1799. Research Diploma, Bournemouth Polytechnic (now University), Bournemouth.

Hudson B. (1986) Lessons from the Jasmine Beckford inquiry. *Midwife, Health Visitor and Community Nurse*, **22**, 162–163.

Jorgenson D.L. (1989) *Participant Observation*. Sage, Newbury Park, California.

Josselson R. & Lieblich A. (1993) *The Narrative Study of Lives*. Sage, Newbury Park, California.

Kleinman A. (1988) *The Illness Narratives: Suffering, Healing and the Human Condition*. Basic Books, New York.

LeCompte M.D. & Preissle J. with Tesch R. (1993) *Ethnography and Qualitative Design in Educational Research* 2nd edn. Academic Press, Chicago.

McClelland M. & Sands R.G. (1993) The missing voice in interdisciplinary communication. *Qualitative Health Research*, **3**(1), 74–90.

Malinowski B. (1922) *Argonauts of the Western Pacific: An Account of Native Enterprise and Adventure in the Archipelagoes of Melanesian New Guinea*. Dutton, New York.

Marshall C. & Rossman G.R. (1995) *Designing Qualitative Research* 2nd edn. Sage, Thousand Oaks, California.

May K.A. (1991) Interview techniques in qualitative research. In *Qualitative Nursing Research: A Contemporary Dialogue* (ed. J.M. Morse), pp. 188–209, Sage, Newbury Park, California.

Mead M. (1935) *Sex and Temperament in Three Primitive Societies*. Morrow, New York.

Melia K. (1987) *Learning and Working*. Tavistock, London.

Merriam S.J. (1988) *Case Study Research in Education*. Jossey Bass, San Francisco.

Nettleton S. & Harding G. (1994) Protesting patients: a study of complaints submitted to a Family Health Service Authority. *Sociology of Health and Illness*, **16**(1), 38–61.

Patton M. (1990) *Qualitative Evaluation and Research Methods*. Sage, Newbury Park, California.

Platt J. (1981) On interviewing one's peers. *British Journal of Sociology*, **32**(1), 75–91.

Riessman C.K. (1993) *Narrative Analysis*. Sage, Newbury Park, California.

Robinson I. (1990) Personal narratives, social carers and medical courses: analysing trajectories in autobiographies of people with multiple sclerosis. *Social Science and Medicine*, **30**(11), 1173–1184.

Rosenhan D.L. (1973) On being sane in insane places. *Science*, **1**(179) 250–258.

Roth J.A. (1963) *Timetables*. Bobbs Merril, Indianapolis.

Scott J. (1990) *A Matter of Record: Documentary Sources in Social Research*. Polity Press, Cambridge.

Seibold C., Richards L. & Simon D. (1994) Feminist method and qualitative research about midlife. *Journal of Advanced Nursing*, **19**, 394–402.

Seidman I.E. (1991) *Interviewing as Qualitative Research*. Teachers College, Columbia

University, New York.

Spradley J.P. (1970) *You Owe Yourself a Drunk: An Ethnography of Urban Nomads.* Little, Brown, Boston.

Spradley J.P. (1979) *The Ethnographic Interview.* Harcourt Brace Janovich, Fort Worth.

Spradley J.P. (1980) *Participant Observation.* Harcourt Brace Janovich, Fort Worth.

Strauss A. L., Schatzman L., Bucher R., Ehrlich D. & Sabshin M. (1964) *Psychiatric Ideologies and Institutions.* Collier MacMillan, London.

Viney L.L. & Bousfield L. (1991) Narrative analysis: a method of psychosocial research for Aids-affected people. *Social Science and Medicine,* **32**(7), 757–765.

Wheeler S.J. (1989) Health visitors' and social workers' perceptions of child abuse. Unpublished BSc dissertation, Bournemouth University, Bournemouth.

Chapter 5

Sampling

The chapter will focus on:

- Sampling parameters
- Purposeful sampling
- Sample size
- Naming the participants

Qualitative approaches demand different sampling techniques than the randomly selected and probabilistic sampling which quantitative researchers often use. The aim of sampling in qualitative research is not only to sample populations; a sample consists of sampling units which can be people, concepts, time or setting. Nurse researchers have to choose whom to sample, what to sample and where to sample, because they cannot investigate everything. It must be remembered that the people and places must be available and accessible. The sampling strategies adopted can make a difference to the whole study. The rules of qualitative sampling are less rigid than those of quantitative methods where a strict sampling frame is established before the research starts.

Morse (1991a) advises that sampling be both appropriate and adequate. Appropriateness means that the method of sampling fits the aim of the study and helps the understanding of the research problem. A sampling strategy is adequate if it generates adequate and relevant information and sufficient quality data.

Sampling takes place after the research focus has been decided. Although qualitative researchers start selecting participants at this stage, they continue the selection throughout the study if more are needed, because emerging ideas are more important than individual people. It is not necessary to specify the overall sample and give an exact number of informants from the beginning of the study, although an initial sample should be given. This sampling strategy differs from quantitative research where all respondents are chosen before the project begins. A qualitative proposal should state, for instance, that the initial sample should consist of x (number of) informants.

Sampling parameters

The investigators not only make decisions about the participants in their study but also about the time and location of the research. Whatever the sample, the criteria for selecting it must be clearly identified.

Sampling parameters do not only involve people (e.g. infection control nurses), processes (e.g. interactions between nurses and patients), events (e.g. entry to a hospital ward) and activities (e.g. giving injections and taking blood pressure) as Miles & Huberman (1994) suggest; specific times can also be chosen for sampling (such as morning and afternoon or 6 months before and after visiting a pain clinic).

Example 1 *Settings*

A nurse has decided that he wants to study patients' adherence to medical and nursing advice. His initial sample is patients from a surgical ward. He is interested in whether similar data could be collected from patients in a medical ward and therefore researches people in this setting.

Example 2 *Time*

A researcher finds that patients are restless at a particular time of the morning. She might then focus on a specific time in the afternoon to see whether patients behave in a similar way at that time.

Purposeful (or purposive) sampling

Patton (1990) states that the underlying principle of gaining rich, in-depth information guides the sampling strategies of the qualitative researcher. The selection of participants, settings or units of time must be criterion-based, that is, certain criteria are applied, and the sample is chosen accordingly. Sampling units are selected for a previously specified purpose, therefore the term 'purposive' or 'purposeful' sampling is used. LeCompte & Preissle (1993) assert that criterion-based is a better term for this type of sampling than purposive, because most sampling strategies, even random sampling, are highly purposive. However, the latter is the term used by most researchers.

Researchers must ask two questions: what to sample and how to sample. People generally form the main sampling units. The useful informant is chosen by the researcher or may be self-selected. Sometimes researchers can easily identify individuals or groups with special knowledge of a topic; occasionally they advertise or ask for informants who have insight into a particular situation or are experts in an area of knowledge. For example, they could be nurses who have cared for people undergoing analysis or patients who have had day surgery. Identification of a particular population provides boundaries between those who are included in the study and those who stay outside it. The members of the sample share certain characteristics.

Useful informants would be people who have undergone or are undergoing experiences about which the researcher wants to gain information. For example, individuals who have had a heart transplant might share experiences and the meanings which these have for them with the nurse researcher.

Informants with special knowledge or experience include newcomers, or those who are changing status in a setting. Individuals who are willing to talk about their experience and perceptions are often those persons who have a special approach to their work. Some have power or status, others are naive, frustrated, hostile or attention seeking, although one must remember that these are not always the best informants because they may have a mainly negative perception of the organisation or institution which they discuss. The sample might include people who have lost power and are frustrated, or those that are not jeopardised by uncovering their own practices and ideologies. Morse (1991b:132) identifies the good informant: 'Good informants must be willing and able to critically examine the experience and their response to the situation ... must be willing to share the experience with the interviewer'.

Sampling types

There are a number of different types of sample and sampling. We shall discuss only the following, because they are the most often used and important types of sampling. (An overview of a whole range can be found in Patton (1990) and Kuzel (1992), although many sampling types overlap.)

- Homogeneous sample
- Heterogeneous sample
- Total population sample
- Chain referral sampling
- Convenience or opportunistic sample
- Theoretical sampling

A *homogeneous sample* consists of individuals who belong to the same subculture or have similar characteristics. Nurses often use homogeneous sample units when they wish to observe or interview a particular group, for instance specialist nurses. Midwives may wish to examine attitudes of community midwives. In the preceding cases, a homogeneous group is being studied. The sample can be homogeneous with respect to a certain variable only, for instance occupation, length of experience, type of experience, age or gender. The important variable could be established before the sampling starts.

A *heterogeneous sample* contains individuals or groups of individuals who differ from each other in a major aspect. For instance, nurses may wish to explore the perceptions of RGNs, ENs and auxiliaries who care for patients with HIV. The three groups form a heterogeneous sample. Heterogeneous sampling is also called maximum variation sampling (Patton 1990, Kuzel 1992) because it involves a search for variations in settings and for individuals with widely differing experiences.

> ### Example
>
> A very good example can be found in an ethnographic study by Tarasuk &
> Eakin (1995). These researchers investigated the link between work-related
> back injury and moral judgments that were made by others. The hetero-
> geneous sample consisted of males and females, across a broad range of ages,
> who had different jobs and came from a variety of different backgrounds.
> This was done to maximise contrasts between the participants.

May (1991) suggests that the initial sample might consist of a natural group, while
later sampling is based on early findings with this group and cannot be determined
prior to the study. For instance, a midwife could sample women who have just
given birth to their first child and find that it would be interesting to select older
and younger primiparae because they might have different ideas about childbirth.
Sometimes married couples are chosen as samples or people who live together.
Occasionally the sample consists of focus groups, for instance self-help groups.

A variation of purposive sampling is *snowball or chain referral sampling* (Biernacki
& Waldorf, 1981). Morse (1991a) calls this type 'nominated sampling'. A previously
chosen informant is asked to suggest other individuals with knowledge of a particular area or topic, who participate and in turn nominate other individuals for the
research. Researchers use snowball sampling in studies where they cannot identify
useful informants, where informants are not easily accessible or where anonymity is
desirable, for instance in studies about drug addiction or alcohol use.

> ### Example
>
> Three American researchers, Kearney and her colleagues (1994), interviewed
> women who used crack about sexuality and reproductive issues. Instead of
> accessing these women directly, the researchers preferred chain referral
> sampling.

Morse (1991a) mentions a *total population sample* when all participants selected
come from a particular group. For instance, all the nurses with specific knowledge
or a skill, such as counselling, might be interviewed because the researcher focuses
on this skill, and there might be few available with this skill. All midwives in one
midwifery unit might be interviewed because not only could the experiences of
midwives be important but also the specific setting in which they work, or the
special techniques they adopt.

LeCompte & Preissle (1993) identify other methods of purposeful or criterion-
based sampling:

- Extreme-case selection
- Typical-case selection
- Unique-case selection

In extreme case selection, the researcher identifies certain characteristics for the setting or population. Then extremes of these characteristics are sought and arranged on a continuum. The cases that belong at the two ends of this continuum become the extreme cases. For instance, nurses may study a very large or a very small ward. These can be compared with those which are the norm for the population.

In typical case selection researchers create a profile of characteristics for an average case and find instances of this. They might exclude the very young or old, the almost healthy and the most vulnerable, or any other participants at the end of the continuum.

When choosing unique cases, researchers study those that differ from others by a single characteristic or dimension, such as people who share a particular condition but come from an unusual community, such as a sect or ethnic group.

The terms *convenience* or *opportunistic* sampling are self-explanatory. The researcher uses opportunities to ask people who might be useful for the study. To some extent, of course, most sampling is opportunistic and arranged for the convenience of the researcher. This sometimes happens when recruiting people is difficult.

Example

Bach & McDaniel (1995), who conducted interviews with quadriplegic people in the community, used posters in living centres, or access offices of colleges or universities, to find the sample.

Glaser & Strauss (1967) advocate *theoretical sampling* in the process of collecting data. Theoretical sampling develops as the study proceeds, and it cannot be planned beforehand. Researchers select their sample on the basis of concepts and theoretical issues which arise during the research. The theoretical ideas control the collection of data; therefore researchers have to justify the inclusion of particular sampling units. (Theoretical sampling will be discussed in more detail in Chapter 7.) At the point of data saturation, when no new ideas arise, sampling can stop.

Kuzel (1992) lists five important characteristics of sampling in qualitative research:

(1) Flexible sampling which develops during the study
(2) Sequential selection of sampling units
(3) Sampling guided by theoretical development which becomes progressively more focused
(4) Continuing sampling until no new relevant data arise
(5) Searching for negative or deviant cases

Sample size

The sample may be small or large, depending on the type of research question, material and time resources, as well as on the number of researchers. Generally, qualitative sampling consists of small sampling units studied in depth. Patton (1990) insists that no guidelines exist for sample size in qualitative research, and Benner (1984), for instance, uses a very large heterogeneous sample (109 participants, but these are not all interviewed individually) in her study on nurses and their ideas about caring.

Although there are no rigid rules, research texts often mention that 6–8 data units are needed when the sample consists of a homogeneous group, while 12–20 suffice for a heterogeneous sample (Kuzel, 1992). Most often, the sample consists of between four and 40 informants, though certain research projects contain as many as 200 participants. Qualitative studies which include a large sample size do exist. Sample size, however, does not necessarily determine the importance of the study.

> ## Examples
>
> Field's (1983) sampling frame contained four informants, while Melia (1987) interviewed 40. Strong (1979) included as many as 1000.

We do not see justification for a very large sample in qualitative research. Students or experienced researchers often use these to appease funding bodies which are used to large samples, or research committees which do not know much about qualitative research. Wolcott (1994) asserts that the wish for a large sample size is rooted in quantitative research, where there is a need to generalise. He maintains that a large sample in qualitative research does not enhance the research, indeed it can do harm as it might lack the depth and richness of a smaller sample. Banister *et al.* (1994) claim that when the sample size is too large, the specific response of the participants and their meanings might be lost or not respected.

What shall we call the people we sample?

It is difficult for researchers to know what term to use for the people they interview and observe, especially as this name makes explicit the stance of the researchers and their relationship to those being studied. We favour the terms participant or informant. In surveys, both by structured interviews and written questionnaires, the most frequent term has been respondents, and indeed, many qualitative researchers and research texts still use it (for instance Miles & Huberman, 1994), but it seems less frequent now in nursing research texts and reports.

Morse (1991b) claims that 'respondent' implies a passive response to a stimulus – the researcher's question. It sounds mechanistic. Experimental researchers refer to subjects, again a word that expresses passivity of the people we study. Seidman (1991) argues that this term distinguishes between people as objects and subjects and can be positive, but it also demonstrates inequality between researcher and researched. One might suggest that in qualitative observation studies, this term could be acceptable, but in research with in-depth interviews, it would be inappropriate. 'Interviewee' sounds clumsy and boring.

Anthropologists refer to informants, those members of a culture or group who voluntarily inform the researcher about their world and play an active part in the research. Morse usually chooses this term, though she acknowledges the suggestion by some journal editors that it might be seen to have links to the word 'informant' as used by the police. Most qualitative researchers prefer the term participant, which expresses the collaboration between the researcher and the researched (DePoy & Gitlin, 1993) and the equality of their relationship, but this term may be misleading as the researcher, too, is a participant.

In the end, however, the nurses or midwives must choose for themselves which term suits their research. In Morse's words: 'Subjects, respondents, informants, participants – choose your own term, but choose a term that fits' (Morse, 1991b: 406). We advise our students to use the terms informant or, better still, participant.

Summary

Researchers use sampling procedures which differ from those in quantitative research. There are a variety of sampling types, all purposeful; that is, they are chosen specifically for the study and are criterion-based. The sample of individuals in qualitative research is generally small. Sample units can consist of people, time, setting, processes or concepts (the latter is called theoretical sampling). Sampling is not wholly determined prior to the study but proceeds throughout. The individuals in the study are usually called participants or informants.

References

Bach C.A. & McDaniel R.W. (1995) Techniques for conducting research with quadriplegic adults residing in the community. *Qualitative Health Research*, 5(2), 250–255.

Banister P., Burman E., Parker I., Taylor M. & Tindall C. (1994) *Qualitative Methods in Psychology: A Research Guide*. Open University Press, Milton Keynes.

Benner P. (1984) *From Novice to Expert*. Addison-Wesley, Menlo Park, California.

Biernacki P. & Waldorf D. (1981) Snowball sampling: problems and techniques of chain referral sampling. *Sociological Methods and Research*, 10(2) 141–163.

DePoy E. & Gitlin L.N. (1993) *Introduction to Research: Multiple Strategies for Health and Human Services*. Mosby, St Louis.

Field P.A. (1983) An ethnography: four public health nurses' perspectives on nursing. *Journal of Advanced Nursing*, 8, 3–12.

Glaser B. & Strauss A. (1967) *The Discovery of Grounded Theory*. Aldine, Chicago.

Hammersley M. & Atkinson P.A. (1995) *Ethnography: Principles in Practice* 2nd edn. Tavistock, London.

Kearney M.H., Murphy S. & Rosenbaum M. (1994) Learning by losing: sex and fertility on crack cocaine. *Qualitative Health Research*, **4**(2), 142–185.

Kuzel A.J. (1992) Sampling in qualitative inquiry. In *Doing Qualitative Research* (eds B.F. Crabtree & W.L. Miller), pp. 31–44, Sage, Newbury Park, California.

LeCompte M.D. & Preissle J. with Tesch R. (1993) *Ethnography and Qualitative Design in Educational Research* 2nd edn. Academic Press, Chicago.

May K.A. (1991) Interview techniques in qualitative research: concerns and challenges. In *Qualitative Nursing Research: A Contemporary Dialogue* (ed. J.M. Morse), pp. 188–201, Sage, Newbury Park, California.

Melia K. (1987) *Learning and Working*. Tavistock, London.

Miles M.B. & Huberman A.M. (1994) *Qualitative Data Analysis* 2nd edn. Sage, Thousand Oaks, California.

Morse J. M. (1991a) Strategies for sampling. In *Qualitative Nursing Research: A Contemporary Dialogue* (ed. J.M. Morse), pp. 127–145, Sage, Newbury Park, California.

Morse J. M. (1991b) Subjects, respondents, informants and participants. *Qualitative Health Research*, **1**, 403–406.

Patton M. (1990) *Qualitative Evaluation and Research Methods*. Sage, Newbury Park, California.

Seidman I.E. (1991) *Interviewing as Qualitative Research*. Teachers College, Columbia University, New York.

Strong P.M. (1979) *The Ceremonial Order: Parents, Doctors and Medical Bureaucracies*. Routledge Kegan Paul, London.

Tarasuk V. & Eakin J.M. (1995) The problem of legitimacy in the experience of work-related back injury. *Qualitative Health Research*, **5**(2), 204–221.

Wolcott H.F. 1994 *Transforming Qualitative Data: Description, Analysis, and Interpretation*. Sage, Thousand Oaks, California.

Chapter 6

Ethnography

In this chapter we shall discuss:

- History and origins of ethnography
- The exploration of culture
- The main features of ethnography
- Micro- and macro-ethnographies
- Fieldwork
- Doing and writing ethnography
- Evaluating ethnography

Ethnography is the direct description of a culture or subculture. As the oldest of the qualitative methods, it has been used since ancient times, for instance by the Greeks and Romans who wrote about the cultures which they encountered in their travels and wars. Deriving from the Greek, the term ethnography means a description of the people, literally 'writing of culture' (Atkinson, 1992). It can be distinguished from other forms of qualitative research by its focus on the cultural perspective (Wolcott, 1982). Ethnographic data collection takes place mainly through observations, interviews and examination of documents.

Ethnographers stress the importance of studying human behaviour in the context of a culture in order to gain understanding of the cultural phenomena, rules and norms. Agar (1990) explains that the meaning of ethnography is ambiguous; it refers both to a process – the methods and strategies of research – and to a product – the written story which is the outcome of the research. People 'do' ethnography; they study a culture, observe its members' behaviours and listen to them. They also produce an ethnography, a written text.

Using ethnographic methods, especially observation, helps health professionals to contextualise the behaviour, beliefs and feelings of their clients or colleagues. Through ethnography, nurses and midwives become culturally sensitive and can identify the cultural influences on the individuals and groups they study. The goals of nurse ethnographers, however, differ from those of researchers in a subject discipline such as anthropology or sociology. Hammersley & Atkinson (1995) claim that ethnography aims to produce knowledge rather than improve professional practice, but much ethnography in education, for instance, was intended to improve practice. Nurse ethnographers see the production of knowledge only as a first step; on the basis of this, they seek to improve their nursing practice.

History and origins of ethnography

Modern ethnography has its roots in social anthropology and emerged in particular in the 1920s and 1930s when famous anthropologists such as Malinowski (1922), Boas (1928) and Mead (1935), while searching for cultural patterns and rules, explored a variety of non-western cultures and the life styles of the people within them. After the world wars, when tribal groups were disappearing, researchers wished to preserve aspects of vanishing cultures by living with them and writing about them.

In the beginning these anthropologists explored only 'primitive' cultures (a term which demonstrates the patronising stance of many early anthropologists). When cultures became more linked with each other and western anthropologists could not find homogeneous isolated cultures abroad, they turned to researching their own cultures, acting as 'cultural strangers'. This means trying to see a culture from the outside; everything is looked at with the eyes of an outsider. Sociologists, too, adopted ethnographic methods, immersing themselves in the culture or subculture in which they took an interest. Experienced ethnographers and sociologists who are researching their own society take a new perspective on that which is already familiar. This approach to a familiar culture helps ethnographers not to take assumptions about their own society or cultural group for granted.

The Chicago school of sociology, too, had an influence on later ethnographic methods because its members examined marginal cultural and 'socially strange' subcultures like the slums, ghettos and gangs of the city. A good example is the study by Whyte (1943), who investigated the urban gang subculture in an American city. *Street Corner Society* became a classic, and other sociologists used this work as a model for their own writing.

Culture

Anthropology is concerned with culture. Culture can be defined as the total way of life of a group, the learnt behaviour which is socially constructed and transmitted. The life experiences of members of a cultural group include a communication system which they share. This consists of signs such as gestures, mime and language, as well as cultural artefacts – all messages which the members of a culture recognise, and whose meaning they understand.

Example

Wenger (1985) studied the culture of Soviet Jewish immigrants into the United States and explored their views on health and health care experiences. She gained access to the community, observed and listened, involving key informants who had special knowledge of the group. Wenger arrived at a number of 'cultural themes', ideas that came directly from the immigrant culture.

Individuals in a culture or subculture hold common values and ideas acquired through learning from other members of the group. Goetz & LeCompte (1984) stress the researchers' responsibility to describe the unique and distinctive processes of the subculture or culture they study. Social anthropologists aim to observe and study the modes of life of a culture. This they do through the method of ethnography. They analyse, compare and examine groups and their rules of behaviour. The relationship of individuals to the group and to each other is also explored. The study of change, in particular, helped ethnographers understand cultures and subcultures. In areas where two cultures meet, they focus on the conflict between groups.

Sarantakos (1993) and Thomas (1993) distinguish between two types of ethnographic methods:

- descriptive or conventional ethnography
- critical ethnography

Descriptive or conventional ethnography focuses on the description of cultures or groups and, through analysis, uncovers patterns, typologies and categories. Critical ethnography involves the study of macro-social factors such as power and examines common-sense assumptions and hidden agendas. It is therefore more political. Thomas (1993:4) states the difference: 'Conventional ethnographers study culture for the purpose of describing it; critical ethnographers do so to change it'. (Both kinds of ethnography use the same methods of analysis and will not be discussed separately in this chapter.)

Ethnography in nursing and midwifery

In nursing and midwifery, ethnographic methods were first used in the United States. Some of the best known nursing ethnographers are Leininger (1978, 1985) and Morse (1991, 1994), who have written several well-known texts. Leininger (1985) uses the term *ethnonursing* for the use of ethnography in nursing. She developed this as a modification and extension of ethnography. Ethnonursing deals with studies of a culture like other ethnographic methods, but it is also about nursing care and specifically generates nursing knowledge, 'it is a specific research method focused primarily on documenting, describing and explaining nursing phenomena'.

Muecke (1994) states that differences exist between studies in general anthropology and ethnography in nursing. She considers the goal of nursing ethnography to be more than the understanding of nursing or patient culture, it should lead to an advance in clinical practice. Nurse ethnographers differ from other anthropologists in that they only live with informants in their working day and spend their private lives away from the location where the research takes place. Nurses, of course, are familiar with the language used in the setting, while early anthropologists rarely knew the language of the culture they examined from the beginning of the research, and even modern anthropologists are not always familiar with the setting, the terminology and the people they study.

Ethnographic methods in nursing and midwifery are ways of examining behaviours and perceptions in clinical settings. Ethnographies in this field incorporate studies of health care processes, settings and systems. They include studies of socialisation of nurses or midwives, observations of wards or investigations of patient experiences.

> ## Example
>
> An experienced nurse wished to explore the culture of hospice nurses. From her experience in a hospice at an early stage in her career, she was aware of a difference between hospital and hospice nurses and their perceptions of death and dying. For her study she interviewed hospice and hospital nurses and observed their interactions with dying patients and each other (undergraduate experience).

Nurse ethnographers do not always investigate their own cultural members. In modern Britain nurses care for patients from a variety of ethnic groups and need to be knowledgeable about their cultures. Culture becomes part of all aspects of nursing because both nurses and patients are products of their group. DeSantis (1994) advises that nurses temporarily suspend their own values when dealing with members from other cultures or subcultures. She states that at least three cultures are involved in interaction with patients: the nurse's professional culture, the patient's culture and the context in which the interaction takes place.

The main features of ethnography

The main features of ethnography are

- The collection of data from observation and interviews
- 'Thick' description and the naturalistic stance
- Work with key informants
- The emic/etic dimension

Data collection through observation and interviewing

Researchers collect data by standard methods, mainly through observation and interviewing, but they also rely on documents such as letters, diaries and taped oral histories of people in a particular group or connected with it. Wolcott (1994) calls these strategies *experiencing* (participant observation), *enquiring* (interviewing) and *examining* (studying documents).

As in other qualitative approaches, the researcher is the major research tool. Direct participant observation is the main way of collecting data from the culture under study, and observers try to become part of the culture, taking note of everything they see and hear but also interviewing members of the culture to gain their interpretations.

Health researchers commonly observe behaviour in the clinical or educational setting. Goetz & LeCompte (1984) advise novices not to get lost in detail as it is difficult to describe the social reality of a culture in all its complexity. The decisions about inclusion and exclusion depend on the research topic, the emerging data and the experiences of the researchers. The participants and their actions are observed, and the ways in which they interact with each other, but special events and crises, the site itself and the use of space and time are examined. Observers study the rules of a culture or subculture and the change that occurs over time in the setting. Richardson (1990) warns us that the findings don't just consist of the interviews and fieldnotes; the accounts must be formed into a story, a text which emerges from the data.

Observations become starting points for in-depth interviews. The researchers may not understand what they see, and may ask the members of the group or culture to explain it to them. Participants share their interpretations of events, rules and roles with the interviewer. Some of the interviews are formal and structured, but often researchers ask questions on the spur of the moment, they have informal conversations with members. Often they uncover discrepancies between words and actions, what people do and what they say, a problem discussed by Deutscher (1970). On the other hand there may be congruence between the spoken word and behaviour. Germain (1993) advises that these congruences or discrepancies should be evaluated and explained. All these investigations become part of the ethnographic analysis.

Nurse ethnographers take part in the life of people, they listen to their informants' words and the interpretation of their actions. In essence, this involves a partnership between the investigator and the informants.

The use of thick description

One of the major characteristics of ethnography is thick description, a term used by the anthropologist Geertz (1973), who borrowed it from the philosopher Ryle. It is description which makes explicit the detailed patterns of cultural and social relationships and puts them in context. Ethnographic interpretation cannot be separated from time, place, events and actions of people. It is based on the meaning that actions and events have for the member of a culture. Description and analysis have to be rooted in reality; researchers think and reflect about social events and conduct.

Thick description must be theoretical and analytical in that researchers concern themselves with the abstract and general patterns and traits of social life in a culture. Denzin (1989a) claims that thick description aims to give readers a sense of the emotions, thoughts and perceptions that research participants experience. It deals with the meanings and interpretations of people in a culture.

As stated before, thick description can be contrasted with thin description

(Denzin, 1989a) which is superficial and does not explore the underlying meanings of cultural members. A study where thin description prevails is not a good ethnography.

Selecting key informants and settings

As in other qualitative methods, nurse ethnographers generally use purposive sampling which is criterion-based and non-probabilistic (Goetz & LeCompte, 1984). This means ethnographers adopt certain criteria to choose a specific group and setting to be studied, be it a ward, a group of specialist nurses or patients with a specific condition. Some of our students have used samples from the cultures of recovering alcoholics, patients with myocardial infarction, children with asthma and many other groups. The criteria for sampling must be explicit and systematic (Hammersley & Atkinson, 1983).

Researchers should choose key informants carefully to make sure that they are suitable and representative of the group under study. Leininger (1985) claims that a small sample of key informants can be more useful to the researcher than a large sample of general participants without specific knowledge of a topic. Key actors often participate by informally talking about the cultural conduct or customs of the group. They become active collaborators in the research rather than passive respondents.

The sample is taken from a particular cultural or subcultural group. Ethnographers have to search for individuals within a culture who can give them specific detailed information about the culture. Fetterman (1989) disapproves of the term 'informant' because he sees its origin in colonial settings and linked to 'clandestine activities' which conflict with ethnographic methods. Most ethnographers still use the term and do not perceive it as negative. Key informants own special knowledge about the history and subculture of a group, about interaction processes in it and cultural rules, rituals and language. The key actors help the researcher to become accepted in the culture and subculture. Researchers can validate their own ideas or perceptions with those of key informants by going back to them at the end of the study and asking them to check the script and interpretation (member check).

Example

One of our students examined the thoughts and perceptions of relatives who cared for old people. She chose as her key informants a group of individuals who were part of an informal carers' group. They allowed her to sit in on meetings and listen to their ideas and thoughts, helping her to become acquainted with the subculture of care and also other carers. When she found something that seemed interesting or puzzling to her, she went to the key members of the group for information and eventually for confirmation of her interpretations (undergraduate experience).

The bond between researcher and key informant strengthens when the two spend time with each other. Through informal conversations, researchers can learn about the customs and conduct of the group they study, because key informants have access to areas which researchers cannot reach in time and location. For instance, a midwife might wish to gain information about midwifery during the war, or a nurse wants to discover the problems of nursing abroad, and they have no access themselves to the past or the location. These researchers use informants who have this special knowledge; in these instances midwives who practised during the war or nurses who have extensively worked abroad.

Key informants may be other health professionals or patients. DeSantis (1994) sees patients as the main cultural informants in nursing ethnography. They tell the nurses of their culture or subculture, and of the expectations and health beliefs that form part of it. Spradley (1979) advises ethnographers to elicit the 'tacit' knowledge of cultural members, the concepts and assumptions which they have but of which they are unaware.

Fetterman (1989) warns against prior assumptions which key informants might have. If they are highly knowledgeable they might impose their own ideas on the study and the researcher, therefore the latter must try to compare these tales with the observed reality. There might be the additional danger that key actors might only tell what researchers wish to hear. This danger is particularly strong in the health system. Clients are aware of labelling processes and often want to please those who care for them or deal with them in a professional relationship. However, the lengthy contact of interviewer and informants helps to overcome this.

The emic–etic dimension

Ethnographers use the constructs of the informants and also apply their own scientific conceptual framework, the so-called emic and etic perspectives (Harris, 1976). First, the researcher needs an understanding of the emic perspective, the insider's or native's perceptions. The insider's accounts of reality help to uncover knowledge of the reasons why people act as they do. A researcher who uses the emic perspective gives explanations of events from the cultural member's point of view. This perspective is essential in a study, particularly in the beginning, as it prevents the imposition of the researchers' values and beliefs on to those of another culture.

The outsider's perspective, the etic view, has been prevalent for too long in health care and health research. Outsiders, such as health professionals or professional researchers, used to identify the problems of patients and described them rather than listening to the patients' own ideas. Now, those who experience an illness are allowed to speak for themselves, as they are experts not only on their condition but also on their own feelings and perceptions. As Harris (1976:36) states: 'The way to get inside of people's heads is to talk with them, to ask questions about what they think and feel'. The emic perspective corresponds to the reality and definition of informants.

Researchers who are examining a culture or subculture gain knowledge of the existing rules and patterns from its members; the emic perspective is thus culturally specific. For nurses and midwives who explore their own culture and that of their patients, the 'native' view is not difficult to obtain because they are already closely involved in the culture. This prior involvement can be dangerous though, because health professionals, by being part of the culture they examine, lose awareness of their role as researchers and sometimes rely on assumptions which do not necessarily have a basis in reality. Therefore reflection on prior assumptions is important.

Example

Many patients do not comply with advice from health professionals, who may believe that they don't understand this advice or are deliberately flouting it. By taking the emic perspective on adherence (formerly the term compliance was used) for instance, nurses learn to understand why patients don't follow suggestions and guidelines, or take their medicine when health professionals feel they should. In their research, nurses might find financial, emotional or other personal reasons which have priority for some patients, preventing them from adhering to professional advice.

Of course, the 'etic' view is important too. Etic meanings stress the ideas of ethnographers themselves, their abstract and theoretical view when they distance themselves from the cultural setting and try to make sense of it. Harris (1976) explains that etics are scientific, objective accounts by the researcher, based on that which is directly observable. The researchers place individuals' ideas in a structural framework and interpret it by adopting a social science perspective on the setting. (Our discussion is a simplistic explanation of a very complex and ambiguous term.)

These ideas correspond directly to those of Denzin (1989b) who speaks of first-order and second-order concepts. First-order concepts are those used in the common-sense perspective on everyday life, while second-order concepts are more abstract and imposed by the researcher. For instance, individuals often mention the term *learning the job*, which could be called a first-order concept recognised by people in everyday life. A social scientist would call the same concept *occupational socialisation*, a second-order concept. The two terms show the difference between lay language and academic language.

It must be kept in mind, however, that the emic view cannot be simply translated into an etic perspective. The meaning of the participants differs from scientific interpretations. Researchers move back and forth, from the reality of informants to scientific interpretation, but they must find a balance between involvement in the culture they study and scientific reflections and ideas about the beliefs and practices within that culture. Fetterman (1989) describes this as *iteration*, where researchers revise ideas and build upon previous stages.

Micro- and macro-ethnographies

Micro-ethnographies focus on subcultures or settings such as a single ward or a group of specialist nurses. Fetterman (1989:38) claims that a micro-study is a 'close-up view as if under a microscope of a small social unit or an identifiable activity within the social unit'. Ethnographers select a setting such as a pain clinic, an operating theatre, a labour ward or a GP practice. Field (1983) for instance, writes an ethnography of public health nurses; two of our students examined a mixed gender ward. Most students choose a micro-ethnographic study as it makes fewer demands on their time than macro-ethnography; it seems more immediately relevant to the world of the nurse and the midwife.

There is a continuum between large and small scale studies, macro- and micro-ethnographies. A macro-ethnography examines a larger culture with its institutions, communities and value systems. In nursing and midwifery this will be a hospital, or the nursing culture. The large scope of the study means a long period of time in the setting and often the work of several researchers. Both types of ethnography demand a detailed picture of the community under study as well as similar strategies for data collection and analysis. The type of study depends, of course, on the focus of the investigation and the researchers' own interests.

Ethnographic research can be very useful during changes in a culture. In a changing health care system, nurses sometimes study developments not only in larger settings such as hospitals or the community, but also in the smaller world of wards and theatres. Change, the transition from one stage or one ideology to another, can provide a useful focus for nursing and midwifery research. In Britain, for instance, the document *Changing Childbirth* (Department of Health, 1993) might have made a significant impact on midwifery practice. Whether it has actually changed practices in a local midwifery unit could usefully be evaluated by an observation study. Most units, however, would use a patient survey to find out about this. Small social units are the most appropriate setting for ethnography by health professionals (Boyle, 1994).

Example

Holland (1993) was very interested in ritual in nursing practice. She observed a group of nurses, a cultural group, in a surgical ward setting, to find out whether ritual behaviour was prevalent. She established that rituals and cultural rules existed. They were an outcome of the common values of the group members and helped to create cohesion among them while not adversely affecting patients.

Fieldwork

The term fieldwork is used by ethnographers and other qualitative researchers to describe data collection outside laboratories. Ethnographers gain most of their data through fieldwork, which involves mainly observation and interviewing. They become familiar with the community or group which they want to investigate. Fieldwork in qualitative research means working in the natural setting of the informants, observing them and talking to them over prolonged periods of time. This is necessary so that informants get used to the researcher and behave naturally rather than putting on a performance. The observation of a variety of contexts is important. Spradley (1980:78) provides the following list in order to guide researchers when they observe a situation, although these guidelines cannot be seen as complete or all inclusive.

(1) *Space:* the physical place or places
(2) *Actor:* the people involved
(3) *Activity:* a set of related acts people do
(4) *Object:* the physical things that are present
(5) *Act:* single actions that people do
(6) *Event:* a set of related activities that people carry out
(7) *Time:* the sequencing that takes place over time
(8) *Goal:* the things that people try to accomplish
(9) *Feeling:* the emotions felt and expressed

The initial phase in the field consists of a time for exploration. Nurses and midwives learn about an area of study and become familiar with it. This is not difficult because they are already part of the community and well aware of patient and professional cultures. Acceptance need not be earned because nurses have been part of these cultures, while anthropologists in foreign cultures must achieve entry through learning the ways of the group.

Fieldwork aims to uncover patterns and regularities in a culture which the people living in that community can recognise. Germain (1993) identifies three stages in fieldwork. In the first stage the researchers gain an overview of the culture under study and write notes on their observations. In the second stage researchers start focusing on particular issues. They question the informants on the initial observations. In the third stage researchers realise that saturation has occurred, and they start the process of disengagement.

The best method of data collection in ethnographic research is participant observation, the most complete immersion in a culture. For instance, a nurse who intends to explore the work of a nursing development unit would either be a member of this unit or take part in it in order to observe the practices and reactions of the individuals within.

The ethnographic record: field and analytic notes

Researchers collect data by standard methods, mainly through observing and interviewing but also relying on documents such as letters and diaries and the oral history of people in the culture they study. From the beginning of their research, nurse ethnographers record what goes on in the field – the setting and situation they are studying. This includes noting down fleeting impressions as well as accurate and detailed descriptions of events and behaviour in context. While writing notes and describing what occurs in the situation, ethnographers become reflective and analytic.

Spradley (1979) lists four different types of field notes in ethnography:

- the condensed account
- the expanded account
- the fieldwork journal
- analysis and interpretation notes

Condensed accounts are short descriptions made in the field during data collection, while expanded accounts extend the descriptions and fill in detail. Ethnographers extend the short account as soon as possible after observation or interview if they were unable to record it during data collection. In the field journal ethnographers note their own biases, reactions and problems during fieldwork. Researchers use additional ways to record events and behaviour, such as tapes, films or photographs, flowcharts and diagrams.

Fieldwork proceeds in progressive stages. Initially researchers gain the broad picture of the group and the setting. They observe behaviour and listen to the language which is used in the community they study. For nurses and midwives in a clinical setting this is not difficult because patients, colleagues and other health professionals trust them to record accurately and honestly. After initial observation researchers focus on particular issues which seem important to them. Finally, the writing becomes a detailed analysis and interpretation of the culture under study.

Doing and writing ethnography

Ethnographers start by experiencing, enquiring and examining (Wolcott, 1992). We have discussed these initial procedures. When writing up the research, researchers take all these into account, and they form part of an ethnography. As Wolcott states, an ethnography consists of description, analysis and interpretation. Ethnographers describe what they see and hear while studying a culture; they identify its main features and uncover relationships between them through analysis; they interpret the findings by asking for meaning and inferring it from the data.

Description

'Description – in its everyday sense – is at the heart of qualitative enquiry' says Wolcott (1994:55). We must warn, however, that it is never as simple as it seems. Writers select specific situations for observation, disregard some events and interactions in favour of others and focus on particular issues which they perceive as relevant and significant. Not everything observed or heard is described, but only that which is relevant for the study at hand. This involves at least some analysis and interpretation.

Researchers describe by writing a story which is a report of the actions, inter-actions and events within a cultural group. The reader should get a sense of the setting or 'a feel' for it and understand 'what's going on here'. The description is enhanced by the description of critical events, rituals or roles.

Wolcott demands that during description the writer follows an analytical structure which gives a framework to the account. For instance, nursing students could use chapter headings which reflect the themes arising from the study.

Analysis

Analysis entails working with the data. After processing them by coding, we transform them from the raw data by recognising patterns and themes and making linkages between ideas. Analysis cannot proceed without interpretation but is more scientific and systematic; it brings order to disorderly data, and the researchers must show how they arrived at the structures and linkages. At this stage other people's research connected with the emergent themes becomes part of the analytic process through comparison and integration in the study. It is important that the analysis accurately reflects the data. Whatever the analyst finds has to be related back to the data in order to see whether there is a fit between them and the analytic categories and themes.

Steps in the analysis

As in other qualitative research, data analysis takes place from the beginning of the observation and interviews. The focus becomes progressively clearer. In the data analysis the researcher revisits the aim and the initial research question. Analysis takes more time than data collection. Fielding (1993) claims that in the analysis, description of behaviour and events does not suffice, and that the aim of ethno-graphy is more than the description of a group or a culture. The process of analysis involves several steps:

(1) Ordering and organising the collected material
(2) Re-reading the data
(3) Breaking the material into manageable pieces
(4) Building, comparing and contrasting categories
(5) Searching for relationships and grouping categories together
(6) Recognising and describing patterns, themes and typologies
(7) Interpreting and searching for meaning

Spradley (1979:92) claims that analysis involves the 'systematic examination of something to determine its parts, the relationship among parts, and their rela-tionship to the whole'. Agar (1980) stresses the non-linear nature of the process: researchers collect data through which they learn about a culture; they try to make sense of what they saw and heard, and then they collect new data on the basis of their analysis and interpretation.

The data are scanned and organised from the very beginning of the study. If gaps and inadequacies occur, they can be filled by collecting more data or re-focusing on the initial aims of the study. While this work goes on, researchers choose to focus on particular aspects which they examine more closely than others.

In re-reading the data, thoughts and observations can be recorded, and a search for regularities can begin. The first interview, or the first detailed description of observation, is scanned and marked off into sections which are then given codes. The second and third interview transcripts are then coded and compared with the first. Commonalities and similar codes are sorted and grouped together. This happens for each interview (or observation). Thematically similar sets are placed together. The researcher then tries to find the ideas which link the categories and describes and summarises them. From this stage onwards diagrams are helpful because they present the links and patterns graphically. (The text by Miles & Huberman (1994) is the classic example of the use of diagrams in qualitative research.)

The regularities and emerging themes are grouped into categories which the researcher compares and reduces to major constructs. Broad patterns of thought and behaviour emerge. The patterns and regularities have their basis in the actual observations and interviews; they will be connected with the personal experiences of the researcher and the categories and themes drawn from the literature. Goetz & LeCompte (1984) advise occasional written summaries as useful organising devices.

Interpretation

Researchers take the last step, that of interpretation during and after the analysis, making inferences, providing meaning and giving explanations for the phenomena. While describing and analysing, we interpret the findings, that is, we gain insight and give meaning to them. Interpretation, although linked to the analysis, is not as factual; it is more speculative, involving theorising and explaining. Interpretation links the emerging ideas derived from the analysis to established theories, through comparing and contrasting others' work with one's own.

Eventually the story is put together from the descriptions, analyses and interpretations. LeCompte & Preissle (1993) compare this to assembling a jigsaw puzzle, where a frame is quickly outlined and small puzzle pieces are collected together and placed in position within the frame. The difference is that one knows about the final picture of a jigsaw and has something to work towards, while in qualitative research one merely has an emerging picture whose outline one can only imagine, and which may change in the process of assembly.

Critical notes

There are a number of problems with ethnographic research in the nursing and midwifery culture. First, it is difficult to examine one's own group and become a 'cultural stranger' questioning the assumptions of the familiar culture whose rules and norms have been internalised. Vigilance and advice from outsiders are very important. Secondly, because health professionals often have a background in the natural sciences and are taught to adopt a systematic approach to their clinical work, they sometimes may find it difficult to suffer ambiguity. It is better, however, to admit to uncertainty than to make unwarranted claims about the research. It resembles nursing diagnosis: signs and symptoms are examined for meaning but should never become once-and-for-all interpretations. Findings can be re-interpreted at a later stage in the light of reflection or new evidence.

Our students often write up their research, making statements which seem to be applicable to a whole range of similar situations. An ethnography, like other qualitative research, cannot simply be generalised. Findings from one subculture or one setting are not automatically applicable to other settings. However, Wolcott (1994) asserts that there is always a possibility for generalisation, and often the readers can themselves make that leap. The researcher can make comparisons with other specific situations similar to the case studied and can achieve typicality.

Inexperienced researchers are often too descriptive and present raw data without analysis and interpretation. Even the quotes in the study are not raw data but should have gone through the process of analysis. Nevertheless, at the start of a research career, it is advisable to give more descriptive detail, clear analysis and to be careful with interpretation. With experience the balance might change. It is interesting that on revisiting the work at a later stage, many researchers start re-interpreting the data.

Evaluating ethnography

Leininger (1994) establishes evaluation criteria for qualitative research, which, she claims, should be different in type and language from those for quantitative studies. These criteria can be applied to ethnographies and are summarised below.

(1) *Credibility*. Are the findings believable? Do they represent the 'real' world of the participants?

(2) *Confirmability*. Is all evidence documented and the audit trail established? Have member checks (checks with informants at the end of the interview and study) been made?

(3) *Meaning-in-context*. Have informants been studied in context? Is account taken of their environment and the total situation?

(4) *Recurrent patterning*. Do the patterns which are uncovered re-occur and repeat themselves over time?

(5) *Saturation*. Did the researchers immerse themselves in the phenomena which they have explored? Does the study show thick description? Has it gone so far that no further explanations and interpretations can be found?

(6) *Transferability*. Can the findings from this study be transferred to a similar context or situation under similar conditions?

Leininger (1994) suggests that these six criteria can be used for the evaluation of all qualitative methods, although their importance differs in particular approaches. In ethnography, it is of major importance to find the *emic* truth, the world as experienced by informants. This needs *cultural knowledge and sensitivity* on behalf of the researcher.

Summary

Ethnographers immerse themselves in the culture or subculture they study and try to see the world from the culture members' point of view. Data are collected through participant observation and interviews with key informants. Researchers observe the rules and rituals in the culture and try to understand the meaning and interpretation which informants give to them. They compare these with their own *etic* view and explore the differences between the two. Field notes are written throughout the fieldwork about events and behaviour in the setting. Ethnographers describe, analyse and interpret the culture and the local, emic perspective of its members.

After the data have been collected and analysed, researchers write a detailed and lively story: a micro-ethnography, where the focus is on a small setting, or a macro-ethnography, which deals with a larger culture. The main evaluative criterion is the way in which the study presents the culture as experienced by its members.

References

Agar M. (1980) *The Professional Stranger: An Informal Introduction to Ethnography*. Sage, Newbury Park, California.

Agar M. (1990) Exploring the excluded middle. *Journal of Contemporary Ethnography*, **19**(1) (special issue: The Presentation of Ethnographic Research), 73–88.

Atkinson P. (1992) *Understanding Ethnographic Texts*. Sage, Newbury Park, California.

Boas F. (1928) *Anthropology and Modern Life*. Norton, New York.

Boyle J.S. (1994) Styles of ethnography. In *Critical Issues in Qualitative Research Methods* (ed. J.M. Morse), pp. 159–185, Sage, Thousand Oaks, California.

Denzin N.K. (1989a) *The Research Act: The Theoretical Introduction to Sociological Methods* 3rd edn. Prentice Hall, Englewood Cliffs, NJ.

Denzin N.K. (1989b) *Interpretive Interactionism*. Sage, Newbury Park, California.

Department of Health (1993) *Report of the Expert Maternity Group (Changing Childbirth)*. HMSO, London.

DeSantis L. (1994) Making anthropology clinically relevant to nursing care. *Journal of Advanced Nursing*, **20**, 707–715.

Deutscher I. (1970) Words and deeds: social science and social policy. In *Qualitative Methodology: Firsthand Involvement with the Social World* (ed. W.J. Filstead), pp. 27–51, Markham, Chicago.

Fetterman D.M. (1989) *Ethnography: Step by Step*. Sage, Newbury Park, California.

Field P.A. (1983) An ethnography: four public health nurses' perspectives on nursing. *Journal of Advanced Nursing*, **8**, 3–12.

Fielding N. (1993) Ethnography. In *Researching Social Life* (ed. N. Gilbert), pp. 154–171, Sage, Newbury Park, California.

Geertz C. (1973) *The Interpretation of Cultures*. Basic Books, New York.

Germain C.P. (1993) Ethnography: the method. In *Nursing Research: A Qualitative Perspective* 2nd edn (eds P.L. Munhall and C. Oiler Boyd), pp. 237–267, National League for Nursing Press, New York.

Goetz J.P. & LeCompte M.D. (1984) *Ethnography and Qualitative Design in Educational Research*. Academic Press, Orlando.

Hammersley M. & Atkinson P. (1983) *Ethnography: Principles in Practice*. Tavistock, London.

Hammersley M. & Atkinson P. (1995) *Ethnography: Principles in Practice* 2nd edn. Tavistock, London.

Harris M. (1976) History and significance of the emic/etic distinction. *Annual Review of Anthropology*, **5**, 329–350.

Holland C.K. (1993) An ethnographic study of nursing culture as an exploration for determining the existence of a system of ritual. *Journal of Advanced Nursing*, **18**, 1461–1470.

LeCompte M.D. & Preissle J. with Tesch R. (1993) *Ethnography and Qualitative Design in Educational Research* 2nd edn. Academic Press, Chicago.

Leininger M. (1978) *Transcultural Nursing: Concepts, Theories and Practice*. John Wiley & Sons, New York.

Leininger M. (1985) *Qualitative Research Methods in Nursing*. W.B. Saunders, Philadelphia.

Leininger M. (1994) Evaluation criteria and critique of qualitative research studies. In *Critical Issues in Qualitative Research Methods* (ed. J.M. Morse), pp. 95–115, Sage, Thousand Oaks, California.

Malinowski B. (1922) *Argonauts of the Western Pacific: An Account of Native Enterprise and Adventure in the Archipelagoes of Melanesian New Guinea*. Dutton, New York.

Mead M. (1935) *Sex and Temperament in Three Primitive Societies*. Morrow, New York.

Miles M.B. & Huberman A.M. (1994) *Qualitative Data Analysis* 2nd edn. Sage, Thousand Oaks, California.

Morse J.M. (1991) *Qualitative Nursing Research: A Contemporary Dialogue*. Sage, Newbury Park, California.

Morse J. M. (1994) *Critical Issues in Qualitative Research Methods*. Sage, Thousand Oaks, California.

Muecke M. (1994) On the evaluation of ethnographies. In *Critical Issues in Qualitative Research Methods* (ed. J.M. Morse), pp. 187–209, Sage, Thousand Oaks, California.

Richardson L. (1990) Narrative and sociology. *Journal of Contemporary Ethnography*, **19**(1), 116–135.

Sarantakos S. (1993) *Social Research*. Macmillan Press, Basingstoke.

Spradley J.P. (1979) *The Ethnographic Interview*. Harcourt Brace Janovich, Fort Worth.

Spradley J.P. (1980) *Participant Observation*. Harcourt Brace Janovich, Fort Worth.

Thomas J. (1993) *Doing Critical Ethnography*. Sage, Newbury Park, California.

Wenger A.F.Z. (1985) Learning to do a mini ethnonursing research study: a doctoral student's experience. In *Qualitative Research Methods in Nursing* (ed. M. Leininger), pp. 283–316, Grune and Stratton, New York.

Whyte W.F. (1943) *Street Corner Society: The Social Structure of an Italian Slum*. University of Chicago Press, Chicago.

Wolcott H. (1982) Differing styles of on-site research: or 'if it isn't ethnography, what is it?' *Review Journal of Philosophy and Social Science*, **7**(1,2), 154–169.

Wolcott H. (1992) Posturing in qualitative enquiry. In *Handbook of Qualitative Research in Education* (eds M. LeCompte, W.L. Millroy & J. Preissle), pp. 121–152, Academic Press, San Diego, California.

Wolcott H.F. (1994) *Transforming Qualitative Data: Description, Analysis, and Interpretation*. Sage, Thousand Oaks, California.

Chapter 7

Grounded Theory

In this chapter we aim to describe and explain:

- History and origin
- The main features of grounded theory
- Data collection
- Analytic procedures
- Problems and pitfalls
- Glaser's critique of Strauss and Corbin

One of the major qualitative approaches which has been used by health professionals since the 1960s is grounded theory. Although it has its origins in sociology, grounded theory can be used in any field of study, be it psychology, health or business studies, and for any type of unstructured material, such as interview transcripts, observations or documents. Glaser (1992) claims that grounded theory methods are not specific to a particular discipline or type of data collection. It seems to be particularly useful for health professionals as it is systematic and detailed. Strauss (1987) maintained that it is not a particular technique but 'a style of doing qualitative analysis' with distinct characteristics.

Grounded theory is more structured than other forms of qualitative research, although it uses generally similar approaches to data collection and analysis. It is sometimes suggested that qualitative methods produce descriptive studies. Strauss & Corbin (1990) firmly deny this. They state that a grounded theory must not just be descriptive but should have explanatory power.

History and origin

Grounded theory (GT) was first used in the 1960s by Barney Glaser and Anselm Strauss, two sociologists who worked together on research about health professionals' interaction with dying patients. This generated two books (Glaser & Strauss, 1965, 1968) which have become exemplars for grounded theory. From research and teaching, the classic text *The Discovery of Grounded Theory* emerged (Glaser & Strauss, 1967). Four other books on grounded theory followed: *Field Research: Strategies for a Natural Sociology* (Schatzman & Strauss, 1973), *Theoretical Sensitivity* (Glaser, 1978), *Qualitative Analysis for Social Scientists* (Strauss, 1987) and *Basics of Qualitative Research* (Strauss & Corbin, 1990).

The last book, in which Strauss is co-author with a nurse researcher, is by far the clearest and most practically useful book on grounded theory as it describes an approach which has been tried and clarified over time. It has become particularly fashionable in the last decade and is often used by nurses. A book edited by Chenitz & Swanson (1986) is very good and contains some examples of grounded theory research.

In nursing and health care the grounded theory approach has been popular from its inception, starting with Benoliel's (1973) study on the interaction of nurses with dying patients. Corbin (1987) and Morse (1991) in the USA, Melia (1987) and Smith (1992) in Britain, are some of the nurse researchers who have used this approach. Many nurses have described the techniques and procedures of grounded theory, for instance Stern (1985), Chenitz & Swanson (1986) and Hutchinson (1986). Wuest (1995) claims that GT is particularly useful in nursing because researchers take account of the findings and act on them after having identified the bases of informants' experiences. It is interesting that nurses seem to like the grounded theory approach. We think that this is due to the orderly and systematic way in which the data are collected and analysed. This, after all, is the way in which health professionals do their work.

Symbolic interactionism

The theoretical framework for grounded theory is derived from the insights of symbolic interactionism, focusing on the processes of interaction between people exploring human behaviour and social roles. Symbolic interactionism explains how individuals attempt to fit their lines of action to those of others (Blumer, 1971), take account of each others' acts, interpret them and re-organise their own behaviour.

Mead (1934), the main proponent of symbolic interactionism, sees the self as a social rather than a psychological phenomenon. Members of society affect the development of a person's social self by their expectations and influence. Initially, individuals model their roles on the important people in their lives, 'significant others'; they learn to act according to others' expectations, thereby shaping their behaviour. Eventually, the individual is able to play a number of social roles simultaneously and can organise the roles taken from the community, the 'generalised other'. Mead compares this to a team game, where members of a team anticipate the behaviour of other players and can therefore play their own role. The observation of these interacting roles is a source of data in grounded theory.

The model of the person in symbolic interactionism is active and creative rather than passive. Individuals plan, project, create actions and revise them. By interpreting each other's behaviour, they choose from a variety of social roles. People share the attitudes and responses to particular situations with members of their group. Hence members of a culture or community analyse the language, appearance and gestures of others and act in accordance with their interpretations. On these perceptions, they base their justifications for conduct which can only be understood in context. Grounded theory therefore stresses the importance of the context in which people function.

Symbolic interactionism focuses on actions and perceptions of individuals and their ideas and intentions. The Thomas theorem states: 'If men (sic) define situations as real, they are real in their consequences', thereby claiming that individual definitions of reality shape perceptions and actions. Participant observation and interviewing trace this proess of 'definition of the situation' (Thomas, 1972).

Denzin (1989) links symbolic interactionism to naturalistic, qualitative research methods by stating that researchers must enter the world of interactive human beings to understand them. By doing this, they see the situation from the perspective of the participants rather than their own. This perspective can be uncovered by interviews and diaries. Qualitative methods suit the theoretical assumptions of symbolic interactionism. As human beings are seen as active and creative, they can be observed in the process of their work and their negotiations with others, particularly with significant others. The interpretation of participants in the situation should be heard. Researchers use grounded theory to investigate these interactions, behaviours and experiences as well as individuals' perceptions and thoughts about them.

The main features of grounded theory

One of the main features of grounded theory is the generation of theory from the data, although existing theories can be modified or extended through this method. It emphasises the development of ideas from the data like other qualitative methods but goes further than these. Grounded theory researchers start with an area of interest, collect the data and allow the relevant ideas to develop, while quantitative research begins with preconceived ideas, theories and hypotheses which are then tested for confirmation. Wiener & Wysmans (1990:12) maintain that the concept of grounded theory is not always understood; theory in this approach means:

> 'identifying the relationship between and among concepts, and presenting a systematic view of the phenomena being examined, in order to explain what is going on'.

According to Strauss & Corbin (1990:23) a good grounded theory has four main criteria: fit, understanding, generality and control. It should be true to real life and it should be clearly understandable to the participants and professionals, who are linked to the area of study. Strauss & Corbin (1990) demand that it be applicable to a variety of similar settings and contexts.

Glaser & Strauss (1967) advise that rigid preconceived ideas prevent development of the research; imposing a framework might block the awareness of major concepts which emerge from the data. Grounded theory helps health professionals to give up their own model of patient care and disease management in order to adopt an alternative perspective based on the perceptions and beliefs of patients. For this they need flexibility and open minds, qualities related to the processes involved in nursing, which demand an open and flexible approach.

> Example
>
> Orona (1990) examined the experience of care-giving by relatives of people
> with Alzheimer's disease. The researcher had expected that carers go through
> a process of decision-making before placing their relatives in an institution.
> However, she found that there was no such conscious process, and relatives
> did not focus on decision-making but on the process of identity loss of their
> relative. Identity loss of the person with Alzheimer's disease became the core
> theme. For Orona, the analytic development was not linear or systematic and
> ordered. She needed flexibility to deal with the findings which arose directly
> from the data

Stern (1980) makes a case for grounded theory in situations where little is known
about a particular topic or problem area, or where a new and exciting outlook is
needed in familiar settings.

The grounded theory style of research uses constant comparison. The researcher
compares each section of the data with every other throughout the study for
similarities and differences. Included in this process are the themes and categories
identified in the literature. All the data are coded and categorised, and from this
process major concepts and constructs are formed. The researcher takes up a search
for major themes which link ideas, to find a 'story line' for the study.

The approach is both inductive and deductive. Strauss (1987) sees the processes
of induction, deduction and verification as essential in grounded theory. Grounded
theory does not start with a hypothesis. After collecting the initial data, however,
relationships are established and provisional hypotheses concerned. These are
verified by checking them out against further data. Corbin (1986) reminds the
analyst that this process of grounded theory is very similar to the nursing process
and should prove easy to use for nurses.

Strauss & Corbin (1990) acknowledge that grounded theory has similarities with
other qualitative methods in data sources and emphasis. Grounded theorists accept
their role as interpreters of the data and do not stop at merely reporting them. The
method does, however, differ in that researchers search for relationships between
concepts, while other forms of qualitative research often generate major themes but
do not always uncover patterns and links between categories or develop theories
(see Chapter 14).

Data collection

Data are collected through observations in the field, interviews of participants,
diaries and other documents like letters or even newspapers. Researchers use
interviews and observations more often than other data sources, and they sup-
plement these through literature searches. Indeed, the literature becomes part of
the data that are analysed. Everything, even experiences of researchers, can become

sources of data. Glaser & Strauss (1967) assert that the researcher does not approach the study with an empty mind. In fact, most research is based on prior interest and problems which the researchers have experienced and reflected on, even when there is no hypothesis.

Data collection and analysis are linked from the beginning of the research and proceed in parallel and interact continuously. The analysis starts after the first few steps in the data collection have been taken; the emerging ideas guide the analysis. The gathering of data does not finish until the end of the research because ideas, concepts and new questions continually arise which guide the researcher to new data sources. Researchers collect data from initial interviews or observations and take their cues from the first emerging ideas to develop further interviews and observations. This means that the collection of data becomes more focused and specific as the process develops.

While observing and interviewing, the investigator writes field notes from the beginning of the data collection throughout the project. Certain occurrences in the setting or ideas from the participants that seem of vital interest are recorded either during or immediately after data collection. They remind the researcher of the events, actions and interactions and trigger thinking processes.

Analytic procedures

According to Glaser (1978) the following are necessary for grounded theory:

- Theoretical sensitivity
- Theoretical sampling
- Coding and categorising
- Constant comparison
- The use of the literature as data
- Integration of theory
- Writing theoretical memos and field notes

Theoretical sensitivity

Researchers must be theoretically sensitive (Glaser, 1978). Strauss & Corbin (1990: 42) state that:

> 'theoretical sensitivity refers to the attitude of having insight, the ability to give meaning to data, the capacity to understand and capability to separate the pertinent from that which isn't'.

Indeed, theoretical sensitivity makes the researcher aware of the significance of the data. There are a variety of sources for theoretical sensitivity. It is built up over time, from reading and experience which guide the researcher to examine the data from all sides rather than stay fixed on the obvious.

Professional experience can be one source of awareness, and personal experience, too, can help make the researcher sensitive.

Example 1

An expert nurse explored patient experience in hospital. She knows from her long professional career that patients feel a number of emotions when they first come to hospital. This experience makes her sensitive to patients' feelings and perceptions which she then explores.

Example 2

A midwife was given little information about some aspects of childbirth when she had her first child. She therefore knows, from personal experience, of the problems of lack of information. When she observes or asks questions about the experience of childbirth, she might include questions on the feelings that lack of information can generate.

The literature sensitises in the sense that documents, research studies or autobiographies create awareness in the nurse of relevant and significant elements in the data.

Example

A health professional has read a study about nurses' role learning. He or she might follow up some of the aspects of role learning that are discussed in this study.

Strauss & Corbin (1990) believe that theoretical sensitivity increases gradually when researchers interact with the data, because they think about emerging ideas, ask further questions and see these ideas as provisional until they have been examined over time and are finally confirmed by the data.

Theoretical sampling techniques

Sampling guided by ideas which have significance for the emerging theory is called theoretical sampling. One of the main differences between this and other types of sampling is time and continuance. Unlike other sampling which is planned beforehand, theoretical sampling in grounded theory continues throughout the study and is not planned before the study starts. Wiener & Wysmans (1990:47) reiterate that sampling does not proceed 'in terms of individuals or units of time but in terms of concepts, dimensions and variations'. Theoretical sampling, though originating in grounded theory is occasionally used in other types of qualitative analysis. (Sampling has been discussed in greater detail in Chapter 4.)

At the start of the project, nurses make initial sampling decisions. They decide on a setting and on particular individuals or groups of people able to give information on the topic under study. Once the research has started and initial data have been analysed and examined (one must remember that data collection and analysis interact) new concepts arise, and events and people are chosen who can further illuminate the problem. Researchers then set out to sample different situations, individuals or a variety of settings, and focus on new ideas to extend the emerging theories. The selection of participants, settings, events or documents is a function of developing theories.

Theoretical sampling continues until the point of saturation. Students do not always understand the meaning of the concept *saturation*. They believe that saturation has taken place when a concept is mentioned frequently and is described in similar ways by a number of people, or when the same ideas arise over and over again. This does not necessarily mean that saturation has occurred. Morse suggests that researchers can recognise when saturation has been achieved by the quality of the theory that has been developed: 'saturate data are rich, full and complete' (Morse 1995:149). Saturation occurs at a different stage in each research project and cannot be predicted.

The coding and categorising of data

Coding and categorising goes on throughout the research. From the start of the study, analysts code the data. Coding in grounded theory is the process by which concepts or themes are identified and named during the analysis. Data are transformed and reduced to build categories. Through the emergence of these categories theory can be evolved and integrated.

In this process, the first step is concerned with open coding which starts as soon as the researcher receives the data. Open coding is the process of breaking down and conceptualising the data. Hutchinson (1986) differentiates between level 1, 2 and 3 codes. Level 1 codes are relatively simple. For instance, a novice midwife might describe experiences in hospital: 'I was shocked when I observed the first birth I had ever seen on the ward'. The code for this might be 'initial shock'.

Sometimes these codes consist of words and phrases used by the participants themselves to describe a phenomenon. They are called *in vivo* codes (Strauss, 1987). A new recruit to nursing might declare in an interview: 'I was thrown in at the deep end'. The code might be 'thrown in at the deep end'. *In vivo* codes can give life and interest to the study and can be immediately recognised as reflecting the reality of the participants.

In grounded theory, all the data are coded. Initial codes tend to be provisional and are modified or transformed over the period of analysis. At the beginning of a project or a study, line-by-line analysis is important, although it may be a long drawn-out process for analysts. As codes are based directly on the data, the researcher avoids preconceived ideas. An example of an interview with a nurse tutor gives some idea of level 1 coding

---

Example

Well, I suppose most people get fed up with doing the same things year in year out	People get tired of doing the same thing
I really felt I wanted a change	Wants change
Regular hours seemed important to me	Wants regular hours
I hadn't been promoted to the level which I could function at	Complains of lack of promotion

---

The analyst groups concepts together and develops categories. At the start a great number of labels are used, and after initial coding analysts attempt to condense (or collapse) codes into groups of concepts with similar traits, which are categories. Hutchinson (1986) calls these level 2 codes. These categories tend to be more abstract than initial codes and are generally formulated by the investigator. These are examples of level 2 codes.

Example

I had this fear that I was not going to survive	Fear of dying
Nobody, but nobody was there to help me and I felt that I was completely alone.	Lack of support
We all need somebody close to be with us when we are ill	Need for significant other

---

The broken down data must be linked together again in a new form. The main features (properties) and dimensions of these categories are identified.

Example

Strauss & Corbin (1990:70) use the concept of colour to illustrate this. Properties of colour include intensity, shade, etc., and the distinctions and variations within properties, such as light and dark within a shade of colour, are called dimensions. Dimensions re the places of properties on a continuum (light–dark, high–low, often–never) and they depend on the category and its properties.

Level 3 constructs are major categories which, although generated from the data and based in them, are formulated by the analysts and rooted in their nursing and academic knowledge. These constructs contain developing theoretical ideas and themes, and through building these constructs analysts reassemble the data. Categories are linked to subcategories. This process of reassembling the data is called axial coding. There is no reason why the researcher cannot use the categories that others have discovered. For instance one of our students (Crockford, 1992) used the term 'existential plight' (Weisman & Worden, 1976) to discuss the way the participants of her study, who were nurses, saw the fear and worry of the patients for whom they cared. Melia (1987) takes the term 'awareness context' from Glaser & Strauss (1965).

Although there is no initial hypothesis in grounded theory, during the course of the research working hypotheses are generated. These must be based in and indicated by the data. The process of testing and verification for the hypotheses which link the categories goes on throughout the research. This includes the search for deviant or negative cases which do not support a particular hypothesis. When these are found, the researcher must modify the hypothesis or find reasons why it is not applicable in this particular instance.

The process of coding and categorising only stops when:

(1)   no new information on a category can be found in spite of the attempt to collect more data from a variety of sources
(2)   the category has been described with all its properties, variations and processes
(3)   links between categories are firmly established (Strauss & Corbin, 1990)

The core category

The researcher must discover the core category. In grounded theory, the major category which links all others is called the core category or core variable. Like a thread the category should be woven into the whole of the study and provide the story line. The linking of all categories around a core is called selective coding. This means that the researcher uncovers the essence of the study and integrates all the elements of the emergent theory. The core category is the basic social-psychological process involved in the research (BSP). The BSP is a process which occurs over time and explains changes in behaviour. It demonstrates the ideas that are most significant to the participants.

Example

A project about the perceptions of young people with diabetes shows in essence that they want to be seen as normal by their peers. Thus, 'being normal' may be a core category. On the other hand the study might show that these young people, after discovering diabetes, want to be seen as they were before their illness and try to achieve this by a variety of means. 'Reclaiming a normal self' could be identified as a basic social-psychological process.

Strauss (1987) claims some major characteristics for the core theory:

(1)   It must be the central element of the research, related to other categories and explain variations in behaviour.
(2)   It must recur often in the data and develop as a pattern.
(3)   It is connected with other categories without a major effort by the researcher.
(4)   In the process of identifying, describing and conceptualising the core category, the general theory of the study develops more fully.
(5)   The core category is usually found towards the end of the research.

Coding and categorising involves constant comparison. Initial interviews are analysed and codes and concepts developed. By comparing concepts and sub-categories, researchers are able to group them into major categories and label them. When they code and categorise incoming data, they compare new categories with those that have already been established. Thus, incoming data are checked for their *fit* with existing categories. Each incident of a category is compared with every other incident for similarities and differences. The comparison involves the literature. Constant comparison is useful for finding the properties and dimensions of categories. It helps in looking at concepts critically as each concept is illuminated by the new, incoming data.

The theory

To be credible the theory must have *explanatory power*, linkages between categories and specificity. In a good project, categories are connected with each other and tightly linked to the data. Researchers do not just describe static situations but take into account processes which occur. Glaser & Strauss (1967) state that two types of theory are produced: substantive and formal.

Substantive theory emerges from a study of just one particular context, such as a ward, or patients with myocardial infarction or nurse education, hence this type of theory is very useful for nurses. This type of theory has specificity and applies to the setting and situation studied; this means that it is limited.

Formal theory is generated from many different situations and settings, and is conceptual. It might be a theory about vocational education or about general experiences of suffering. Layder (1993) demonstrates the links between substantive and formal theory. The *career* of the dying patients in hospital, the stages through which they proceed, is substantive theory. When this is linked to the concept of *status passage*, which can be applied to many situations, it becomes formal theory. This type of theory then has general applicability, that is, it holds true not just for the setting of the specific study but also for other settings and situations.

Glaser & Strauss (1967) maintain that grounded theory is superior to the grand theory of the sociologist Talcott Parsons and the middle range theory of Robert Merton. As these latter theories are not rooted in research, they are merely speculative.

Good examples of substantive theory in nursing research are given in the book edited by Morse & Johnson (1991) in which five researchers develop a grounded theory about the illness experience.

> ## Example
>
> A clear example is that given by Johnson (1991). She shows that individuals go through a process of regaining control after a heart attack which is affected by health professionals. Patients test their abilities constantly and adjust until they know that they have again achieved a sense of control.

In a small student project it would be difficult to produce a formal theory with wide applications, but substantive theories can still be important and have general implications for the work of the nurse. Melia (1995), for instance, declares that she meets many nursing students today who recognise their own learning process from her research which traced student socialisation in the late 1970s and 1980s, although this took place in a different system of nurse education.

The literature

The literature becomes a source for data. When categories have been found, researchers trawl the literature for confirmation or refutation of these categories. Analysts try to discover what other researchers have found, and whether there are any links to existing theories. Indeed, the literature becomes part of the data.

Strauss & Corbin (1990) make five main points about the use of the literature.

(1) The literature can stimulate theoretical sensitivity. It can make the analysts aware of ideas which they can check against the data.
(2) The literature becomes part of the data.
(3) The literature can generate questions and problems. Interviews or observations might be illuminated by the literature in which similar or different ideas are discovered. Researchers have to consider why the literature confirms or refutes their ideas.
(4) The literature can guide theoretical sampling. It can help decide where to go next. Ideas might arise which increase the chance of developing further the emerging theory.
(5) The literature can be used to validate the researcher's categories. Concepts in the literature may confirm the findings of the researcher. They may, however, contradict the theory in which case the researcher tries to discover the reasons for this conflict.

Writing field notes and memos

While going through the process of research, the researcher writes field notes and memos. When observing and interviewing, the investigator writes field notes from the beginning of the data collection. Certain occurrences or sentences seem of vital interest and they are recorded either during or immediately after data collection. They remind the researcher of events, actions and interactions and trigger thinking processes. There can be descriptions of the setting.

Example

One of our research students who explored patients' hospital experiences wrote the following when a patient told her that time drags:

Imagine missing something so fundamental. I am too aware of my own busyness to notice the time dragging for patients. Note Roth's classic work is called *Timetables*. (Personal communication, excerpt from field notes, Warren, 1995.)

Strauss & Corbin (1990:197) define memos as 'written records of analysis related to the formulation of theory'. Memos are reports on the analytic progress and should be dated and detailed. Every grounded theory researcher should write memos. They are meant to help in the development and formulation of theory. In theoretical memos the researcher discusses tentative ideas and provisional categories, compares findings and jots down thoughts on the research. Initially, memos might remind the researcher 'don't forget...' or 'I intend to...'; later they encompass micro-codes, and later still, major emergent categories, hunches, implications and concepts from the literature; memos become more varied and theoretical. Ideas for follow-up, related issues and thoughts about deviant cases become part of these memos. Strauss (1987) gives a number of different types of memos; some are preliminary, others are memos on new categories or initial discovery memos. (A complete list is given in Strauss, 1987.)

Example

Strauss (1987:121) demonstrates the use of memos. We shall give an excerpt from a memo which was written during research on hospitals (Strauss *et al.*, 1985): 'Drugs play a large part in comfort work. There are all kinds of drugs for relief of itching, flatulence, constipation, and so on. The array of drugs is immense. Take constipation for example: in the old days, there used to be enemas and a few laxatives. Now there are packaged enema sets, stool softeners, suppositories, laxatives with different chemical reactions. Nurses have to know a lot about what kinds of enemas not to give in certain kinds of illness conditions, forcing fluid intake, etc'.

Strauss (1987) suggests that memos are the written version of an internal dialogue which goes on during the research. Diagrams in the memos can help to remind the analyst and structure the study. Memo-writing continues throughout the whole of the research. It goes through stages and becomes more complex in the process.

Memos and diagrams provide 'density' for the research and guide the researcher 'away from the data to abstract thinking, then in returning to the data to ground these abstractions in reality' (Strauss & Corbin, 1990:199). Eventually, memos become integrated in the writing.

Problems and pitfalls

Writers identify some of the problems of GT. Becker (1993) suggests that some of the studies which use this approach seem too descriptive. Researchers produce good stories including categories or types but often neglect the underlying social processes and abstract concepts. She stresses the need for qualitative researchers to give explanations not just description and this is important particularly in GT. This is echoed by Strauss & Corbin (1994) who emphasise the difference between description and conceptualisation. It is not enough to describe the perspectives of the participant to develop a truly 'grounded' theory.

The terms *emerging categories* and *emerging theory* are criticised by Stern (1994) who maintains that these do not simply 'emerge' as if arising by magic. They have to be worked for and 'pulled' from the data.

Another problem concerns theoretical sampling. Often researchers use selective (or purposive) sampling procedures on which they decide before data collection. For grounded theory research this does not suffice. Theoretical sampling is necessary because of the inductive–deductive nature of the research. Induction is linked to emerging theories which researchers must try to test through theoretical sampling.

Becker (1993) warns the grounded theorist about the use of computers. We know that a number of computer programs for qualitative research exist. Becker feels that computers might prevent sensitivity to the data and the discovery of meanings. Computers distance researchers from the data. Although this need not be so, we realise that in nursing and midwifery research, where emotional engagement and sensitivity is necessary, the use of computers could be problematic.

Generalisability and replicability of grounded theory research are often discussed. It is often suggested that a research project which uses GT is not generally replicable or generalisable. Of course, it is difficult to match the original situation and context. Each researcher has a personal approach and a relationship with the participants which cannot be exactly reproduced. However, if nurses make procedures explicit and clearly describe the original conditions and setting, others can follow the same rules and procedures and discover the same general scheme. Corbin & Strauss (1990) maintain that the findings of a grounded theory study become more generalisable if the study is systematic, and relies on theoretical sampling and examination of special conditions and discrepancies. A range of similar theoretical concepts from a variety of sources can become cumulative.

Glaser's critique of Strauss and Corbin

Stern (1994) distinguishes between two schools of GT which share some common elements but have also major differences. The ideas of Strauss and Glaser seem to have diverged in the last decade. In 1992 Glaser wrote a book in response to Strauss & Corbin's (1990) *Basics of Qualitative Research*, criticising the authors for distorting the procedures and meaning of grounded theory. Glaser claims that the book does not truly describe GT. He accuses the authors of 'forced conceptual description'. The researchers should not impose their research problem but start with an interest and a questioning mind so that they can see their informants' problems with no preconceptions. Thus, the researcher does not start with a research question but with a research interest.

Although agreeing that Strauss and Corbin have described a research method, Glaser (1992) denies that its roots have much in common with the original 1967 volume. The new method, he claims, results in conceptual descriptions rather than in the emergence of concepts and formation of links between them that explain variations in behaviour. The difference between the ideas in Strauss and Corbin's text and the original development lies in the way in which concepts are generated and relationships explained. Glaser argues that participant observation does not suffice for a truly grounded theory; interviews which explain the meanings of the participants are always necessary.

Glaser (1992) believes that any initial literature review would contaminate the data and denies the need for it because it might direct researchers to irrelevant ideas. He had also stated this in his earlier book (Glaser 1978). However, when the concepts are developed the literature can be integrated. Discrepancies between concepts developed from the researchers' original data, the data from the literature may be discovered and the reasons for them investigated. Theoretical sensitivity helps to generate ideas and relate them to theory.

Researchers can make up their own minds which approach to adopt when doing grounded theory. In any case, many researchers adapt methods during the process of research.

Evaluating grounded theory

Strauss & Corbin (1990) claim that GT can be evaluated when the process is made explicit. They developed a number of criteria by which a qualitative study can be judged, and we will summarise these below.

(1)   The selection of the sample and the reasons for this choice
(2)   The description of the major categories
(3)   The indicators on which these categories are based

(4)   The concepts on which theoretical sampling proceeds and their representativeness

(5)   The demonstration of working hypotheses and their confirmation in the data

(6)   An explanation of deviant or negative cases

(7)   The choice of core category and the reasons for the choice

It must be shown that the concepts are grounded in the data, and they should be technical rather than common-sense concepts. The demonstration of systematic links between them becomes important, and these linkages provide the theory which has been generated with 'explanatory power', that is, it should explain variations in the data and identify changes in the process. The link to the phenomenon under study is important, the theoretical ideas which emerged should be significant rather than trivial. This means that they help in understanding the phenomenon and are useful.

Summary

Grounded theory is a style of analysis where data collection and analysis interact. Data usually are collected through non-standardised interviews and observation. Researchers code and categorise transcripts from the data collection, sometimes by using the words of the participants, at other times by using their own interpretive or summarising labels.

The researcher condenses the categories to major constructs, including a core category which provides the link between the categories. Relationships found between categories generate working hypotheses, eventually establishing a new theory. Through this, the storyline emerges. Relevant ideas from the literature and other documents can become part of the data. Throughout the analytic process, constant comparison and theoretical sampling take place. Memos (theoretical notes) provide the researcher with theoretical ideas. The ideas that emerge are thus grounded in the data.

References

Becker P.H. (1993) Common pitfalls in grounded theory research. *Qualitative Health Research*, 3(2), 254–260.

Benoliel J.Q. (1973) *The Nurse and the Dying Patient*. Macmillan, New York.

Blumer H. (1971) Sociological implications of the thoughts of G.H. Mead. In *School and Society* (eds B.R. Cosin *et al.*), pp. 11–17. Open University Press, Milton Keynes.

Chenitz W.C. & Swanson J.M. (1986) *From Practice to Grounded Theory: Qualitative Research in Nursing*. Addison-Wesley, Menlo Park, California.

Corbin J. (1986) Qualitative data analysis for grounded theory. In *From Practice to Grounded Theory: Qualitative Research in Nursing (eds W.C. Chenitz & J.M. Swanson)*, pp. 91–191. *Addison Wesley, Menlo Park, California*.

Corbin J. (1987) Women's perception and management of a pregnancy complicated by chronic illness. *Health Care for Women International*, 84, 317–337.

Corbin J. & Strauss A.L. (1990) Grounded theory research: procedures, canons and evaluative criteria. *Qualitative Sociology*, **13**(1), 3–21.

Crockford E.A. (1992) *Nurses' perceptions of the informational, psychosocial and counselling needs of patients undergoing breast surgery.* Unpublished BSc study, Bournemouth University, Bournemouth.

Denzin N.K. (1989) *The Research Act: A Theoretical Introduction to Sociological Methods* 3rd edn. Prentice Hall, Englewood Cliffs, New Jersey.

Glaser B.G. (1978) *Theoretical Sensitivity.* Sociology Press, Mill Valley, California.

Glaser B.G. (1992) *Basics of Grounded Theory Analysis.* Sociology Press, Mill Valley, California.

Glaser B.G. & Strauss A.L. (1965) *Awareness of Dying.* Aldine, Chicago.

Glaser B.G. & Strauss A.L. (1967) *The Discovery of Grounded Theory.* Aldine, Chicago.

Glaser B.G. & Strauss A.L. (1968) *Time for Dying.* Aldine, Chicago.

Hutchinson (1986) Grounded theory: the method. In *Nursing Research: A Qualitative Perspective* (eds P.L. Munhall & C. Oiler), pp. 111–130. Appleton–Century Crofts, Norwalk, Connecticut.

Johnson J.L. (1991) Learning to live again: the process of adjustment following a heart attack. In *The Illness Experience* (eds J.M. Morse & J.L. Johnson), pp. 13–18. Sage, Newbury Park, California.

Layder D. (1993) *New Strategies in Social Research: An Introduction and Guide.* Polity Press, Cambridge.

Mead G.H. (1934) *Mind, Self and Society.* University of Chicago Press, Chicago.

Melia K. (1987) *Learning and Working.* Tavistock, London.

Melia K. (1995) In a speech given at a Conference on Qualitative Health and Social Care Research, Bournemouth University, Bournemouth, 28–29 September.

Morse J.M. (1991) *Qualitative Nursing Research: A Contemporary Dialogue.* Sage, Newbury Park, California.

Morse J.M. (1995) Editorial. The significance of saturation. *Qualitative Health Research*, **5**(2), 147–149.

Morse J.M. & Johnson J.L. (1991) *The Illness Experience.* Sage, Newbury Park, California.

Orona C.J. (1990) Temporality and identity loss due to Alzheimer's disease. *Social Science and Medicine*, **30**(11), 1247–1256.

Schatzman L. & Strauss A.L. (1973) *Field Research: Strategies for a Natural Sociology.* Prentice Hall, Englewood Cliffs, New Jersey.

Smith P. (1992) *The Emotional Labour of Nursing.* Macmillan, London.

Stern P.N. (1980) Grounded theory methodology: its uses and processes. *Image*, **12**(1), 20–23.

Stern P.N. (1985) Using grounded theory in nursing research. In *Qualitative Research Methods in Nursing* (ed. M. Leininger), pp. 149–160, W.B. Saunders, Philadelphia.

Stern P.N. (1994) Eroding grounded theory. In *Critical Issues in Qualitative Research Methods* (ed. J.M. Morse), pp. 212–223, Sage, Thousand Oaks, California.

Strauss A.L. (1987) *Qualitative Analysis for Social Scientists.* Cambridge University Press, New York.

Strauss A. & Corbin J. (1990) *Basics of Qualitative Research: Grounded Theory Procedures and Techniques.* Sage, Newbury Park, California.

Strauss A. & Corbin J. (1994) Grounded theory methodology: an overview. In *The Handbook of Qualitative Research* (eds N.K. Denzin & Y. Lincoln), pp. 173–285, Sage, Thousand Oaks, California.

Strauss A., Fagerhaugh S., Suczek B. & Wiener C. (1985) *The Social Organization of Medical Work*. University of Chicago Press, Chicago.

Thomas (1972) The definition of the situation. In *Symbolic Interaction* (eds J.G. Manis & B.M. Meltzer), pp. 331–355, Allyn and Bacon, Boston.

Weisman A. & Worden W. (1976) The existential plight in cancer: the significance of the first 100 days. *International Journal of Psychiatry*, 7, 1–15.

Wiener C.L. & Wysmans W.M. (1990) *Grounded Theory in Medical Research*. Swets and Zeitlinger, Amsterdam.

Wuest J. (1995) Feminist grounded theory: an exploration of the congruency and tensions between two traditions in knowledge discovery. *Qualitative Health Research*, 5(1), 125–137.

Chapter 8

Phenomenology: Philosophy and Enquiry

In this chapter we will outline and examine:

- The notion of intentionality and the early stages of phenomenology
- Phases and history of the movement
- Schools of phenomenology
- The research process and procedures for data analysis

Phenomenology, like many words that are unfamiliar, captivates interest, but as a research approach it has often been misunderstood. To address this problem, we have traced the rather complex history of the philosophy of phenomenology and its adaptation as a qualitative research approach. As a method of enquiry it is not often undertaken at undergraduate level but is popular in post-graduate nursing studies. In this chapter we attempt to clarify the process with an example from a study which was directed by the Husserlian School.

The term phenomenology derives from the Greek word *phainein* which means 'to show', 'to be seen', 'to appear' (New Concise Oxford English Dictionary, 1993). Phenomenological philosophy is partly about the ontological question: what is *being*? Ray (1994) claims that it is also connected with the epistemological question (about the theory of knowledge) of 'how we know'.

As philosophy in general, the study of phenomenology is not immediately understandable; Cohen & Omery (1994:136) state that 'phenomenologists are not noted for their clear language'. Nurses, however, have a long experience of tackling jargon from a number of disciplines. Medicine, for instance, is as notorious as any study of the behavioural sciences . Often nurses have to demystify medical language for patients and clients and find other words to describe diseases, investigations and treatments to facilitate patient and client understanding. In general, to understand more fully any new theory, conceptual framework or school of thought, it is useful to trace its origins.

The following section will outline the background of phenomenology from so-called 'continental philosophy', through the subsequent ideas of Franz Brentano and Edmund Husserl, to the later development of the phenomenological movement and schools of phenomenology.

Intentionality and the early stages of phenomenology

Teichman & Evans (1991) describe two different approaches to the study of philosophy, namely *analytic* and *continental*. Analytic philosophy, as the word suggests, is about analysing and defining concepts which are usually abstract. The analytic tradition is the approach used mostly in the United Kingdom and English speaking countries. It is derived originally from the ancient philosophers Socrates, Aristotle and Thomas Aquinas. Continental philosophy, on the other hand, is about taking these abstract concepts and constructing a theory to explain such things as knowledge and existence. It is within this approach to philosophy that phenomenology lies. Continental philosophy, as the name suggests, is mostly found in continental universities. According to Teichman & Evans, it is also practised in South America and parts of the United States.

Phenomenology begins with Edmund Husserl (1859–1938). In the words of Priest (1991:201), Husserl was 'the real initiator of that movement in modern continental philosophy called phenomenology'. It is important, however, to trace the earlier history of phenomenology in the influence of Franz Brentano (1838–1917) on the work of Husserl. This is especially important because Brentano was part of the preparatory phase of this movement (Cohen, 1987).

The central theme of Brentano's philosophy is the notion of intentionality. Intentionality is a way of describing how in consciousness the mind directs its thoughts to an object. Priest describes the notion of intentionality as:

'... the property or characteristic of the mental of being 'of' or 'about' something. For example, it does not make sense to say there is perception but not perception of something or other (even if the perception is an illusion or hallucination). It does not make much sense to talk about there being thinking without there being thinking about something or other (even if what is thought about is imaginary)'.

(Priest 1991:194).

The way Priest describes this feature in Brentano's concept of intentionality is both clear and logical. Yet importantly, he also documents the criticism of this view. Firstly, there may be mental phenomena that are not intentional (i.e. those directed to an object). Secondly, there may be phenomena that are not mental, i.e. physical, but these may be intentional. For the purpose of this chapter, it is not necessary to get involved in this debate. It is important to acknowledge that Husserl was a student of Brentano and influenced by his doctrine of intentionality.

Husserl differed from Brentano, however. Husserl claimed that to state mental phenomena have an intentional object, establishes a relationship between the two. In so doing, questions need to be asked about this relationship. Then three things would arise: the mental act, the intentional object and the relationship. Husserl could not accept that a person is aware of two things at once:

'For example, suppose you are looking at a colour, what you are aware of is colour. You are not aware both of the colour and your awareness of the colour. There are not two items present to your consciousness but only one.'

(Priest 1991:206)

This critical statement concerning Brentano's intentionality shows the complexity of any attempt to define the act of conscious thought. There are many puzzlements concerning the so-called mind–body problem. Philosophers, psychologists and natural scientists, including doctors and psychiatrists, neither agree nor have firmly established what exactly consciousness is, or the true relationship between mind and body. The ideas presented in this chapter cannot resolve the mind–body problem. However, it is useful to note that phenomenology is, in fact, one theory that attempts to do that. Priest places phenomenology within mind–body theories arising from:

(1) Descartes' dualism which separated mind and body.

(2) So called logical behaviourism (which is a belief that everything concerns behaviour: the mind is really observable behaviour).

(3) Notions of idealism (all that exists can be explained in terms of the mind).

(4) Materialism (everything in the universe can be explained in terms of matter).

(5) Functionalism (everything is a kind of cause and effect: the mind is given a stimulus and responds physically or behaviourally).

(6) So called 'double aspect theory' (the physical and mental are, in fact, merely aspects of something else, another reality, outside notions of the mental and the physical).

(7) The phenomenological view (which is an attempt to describe lived experiences without making previous assumptions about the objective reality of those experiences).

Whilst these ideas are presented as theories, Priest points out that phenomenology is, in fact, a practice. It is this practice that is so exciting for nursing, health and social care alike, because it offers the possibility of 'characterizing the contents of experience just as they appear to consciousness with a view to capturing their essential features' (Priest, 1991:183).

Phases and history of the movement

As has already been stated, phenomenology has a philosophical origin. In 1960, Spiegelberg's review of the history of the phenomenological movement was published. He described what he termed three phases in the movement, the preparatory, German and French. Cohen (1987) summarises these in a paper giving her account of the history and importance of phenomenological research for nursing. The influence of Brentano in the so-called preparatory phase has been described above.

The German phase

The German phase involved primarily Edmund Husserl (1859–1938) and later Martin Heidegger (1889–1976). Concerning Husserl's contribution to the movement, Cohen highlights his search for rigour, his criticism of positivism (all knowledge is derived from our senses – linked to scientific enquiry of observation and experiment) and his concepts of *Anschauung* (phenomenological intuiting) and phenomenological reduction. In the former, a different kind of experience is apparent, closely involved with the imagination. Experience suggests a relationship with something real, such as an event, while *Anschauung* can also occur in imagination or memory. The latter is a process which suspends attitudes, beliefs and suppositions in order to properly examine what is present.

Husserl termed this part of phenomenological reduction *epoché* (from the Greek, meaning 'suspension of belief'). There are two stages in this: eidetic reduction and phenomenological reduction proper. Cohen (1987:32) describes the eidetic as the 'reduction from particular facts to general essences'. She points out that bracketing (a mathematical term) is the name given by Husserl to this process of suspending belief. Phenomenological reduction proper is the second stage, and Cohen argues that for researchers this means examining their attitudes, beliefs and prejudices to literally bracket these out, in a sense, remove them from influencing the research (see also Chapter 14). Bracketing and phenomenological reduction are important features of the method, the actual 'doing' of Husserlian phenomenology (these features are identified later in this chapter).

More recently, Koch (1995) has reviewed the influence of Husserl and Heidegger in so-called interpretive research. She argues that Husserl, in fact, maintained Cartesian dualism in his philosophy. For Koch, Husserl's major contribution centred on three features: intentionality, essences and phenomenological reduction (bracketing).

According to Cohen (1987), two important aspects for phenomenology were developed by colleagues and students of Husserl. These are notions of intersubjectivity and the idea of life world (*Lebenswelt*). Intersubjectivity is about the existence of a number of subjectivities which are commonly shared by a community. The concept of life world (*Lebenswelt*) is about the lived experience which is central to modern phenomenology. The idea is that we often do not take into account, or even notice, what is ordinary or common in every day living. Phenomenological enquiry is the approach needed to help to examine and recognise the lived experience which is commonly taken for granted.

The next stage in the German phase of phenomenology involved Heidegger, who was at some point an assistant to Husserl. Due to the recent upsurge of interest (particularly in North America) in using the phenomenological framework for nursing and midwifery research, the work of Heidegger has been examined by Cohen & Omery (1994), Leonard (1994), Ray (1994), Taylor (1994) and Koch (1995). Benner's (1984) phenomenological research uncovered excellence and power in clinical nursing practice, and she references, amongst others, Heidegger. Later Benner & Wrubel (1989) examined and reviewed Heidegger's philosophy.

Taylor (1994) points out that Heidegger's main break from Husserlian phenomenology occurred in the way he developed the notion of *Dasein* which is explained fully in his work *Being and Time* (Heidegger, 1927, and translated into English in 1962). Heidegger's concern was to ask questions about the nature of being. In this sense he was interested in ontological ideas. Ontology, as Teichmann & Evans (1991:2) state 'is the study of the nature of existence and of coming to be'.

Heidegger's notion of *Dasein* is an explanation of the nature of being and existence and as such a concept of personhood.

Leonard (1994) makes five main points concerning a Heideggerian phenomenological view of the person. These are:

(1) The person has a world. (The world comes from culture, history and language. Often this world is so inclusive that it is overlooked and taken for granted until we reflect and analyse.)

(2) The person has a being in which things have value and significance. (In this sense, persons can only be understood by a study of the context of their lives.)

(3) The person is self-interpreting. (A person has the ability to make interpretations about knowledge. The understanding gained becomes part of the self.)

(4) The person is embodied. (This is a different view from the Cartesian, which is about possessing a body. The notion of embodiment is the view that the body is the way we can potentially experience the action of ourselves in the world.).

(5) The person 'is' in time. (This requires a little more elaboration as outlined below.)

Heidegger had a different notion from the one of traditional time which is perceived to flow in a linear fashion, with an awareness of 'now'. According to Leonard (1994) he used the word 'temporality' which denotes a new way of perceiving time in terms of including *the now*, *the no longer* and *the not yet*.

As well as these ideas, Heidegger developed phenomenology into interpretive or hermeneutical methods of enquiry. In classical Greek mythology Hermes was the transmitter of the messages from the Gods to the mortals. This often involved interpreting the messages for the recipients to aid understanding. Hermeneutics developed as a result of translating literature from different languages, or where direct access to authoritative texts, such as the Bible, was difficult. So, according to Bleicher (1980), hermeneutics became the theory of interpretation and developed into its present form as the theory of the interpretation of meaning. Linking this with phenomenology, Koch (1995:831) states:

'Heidegger (1962) declares nothing can be encountered without reference to the person's background understanding, and every encounter entails an interpretation based on the person's background, in its 'historicality'. The framework of interpretation that we use is the foreconception in which we grasp something in advance.'

Heidegger's purpose is going beyond mere description into interpretation (Cohen & Omery, 1994).

The French phase

Cohen (1987) argues that Heidegger's major contribution to the phenomenological movement was his influence on French philosophy. She points out that the main figures in this phase were Gabriel Marcel (1889–1973), Jean Paul Sartre

(1905–1980) and Maurice Merleau Ponty (1908–1961). Marcel did not call himself a phenomenologist but viewed phenomenology as an introduction to analysing the notion of *being*.

Jean Paul Sartre was the most influential figure in the movement but again did not want the label phenomenologist; rather he was described as an 'existentialist'. At this point (if not before) the reader will probably be thinking again about the rather excessive terminology used in philosophy. However, linguistic minefields can be defused in finding a starting point. A useful starting place for this is a dictionary, and we offer a definition of 'existentialism' from *The Chambers Dictionary* (1993) which is as follows:

'A term covering a number of related philosophical doctrines denying objective universal values and holding that people, as moral free agents, must create values for themselves, through actions and must accept the ultimate responsibility for those actions in the seemingly meaningless universe.'

Understanding of terminology can be further enhanced in progression from general to specific. *Collins Dictionary of Philosophy* contains more specific outlines and links existentialism with phenomenology in this passage.

'In so far as existentialist thinking relies heavily on raw experience, it has made use of the work of PHENOMENOLOGY, which attempts to capture experience without imposing on it any prior theoretical views held by the observer. In a purely formal sense, existentialism seeks to emphasise that something is, rather than how it is: the fact of its being, rather than describing the features it has. This has been simply put in the tag that existence comes before ESSENCE. Existence (from Latin *ex(s)istere* to stand out there) is what we have as standing in the world, essence (from Latin *essentia* the being of this or that kind) belongs to a description of us in terms of CONCEPTS.'

(Vesey & Faulkes, 1990:109)

The ideas of existence and essence are from Sartre; his famous and often quoted phrase is 'existence precedes essence'. This is Sartre's idea that a person's actual consciousness and behaviour (existence) comes before character (essence) (Cohen, 1987). In this sense research would focus on real and concrete thoughts and behaviour before imaginary or idealised qualities or essences. The notion of intentionality features also in Sartre's work.

According to Cohen (1987), Merleau Ponty's interest in phenomenology focused on perception and the creation of a science of human being (for the purpose of this chapter it is not necessary to develop this further).

Another major figure in French phenomenology is Paul Ricoeur. Spiegelberg (1971) argues that Ricoeur's phenomenology is primarily descriptive and in fact based upon Husserlian eidetic concerned with essential structures. There are then different approaches within the phenomenological interpretative style. Walters (1995) points out that phenomenology does not have homogeneity. In the next stage of this chapter, we will examine so-called schools of phenomenology outlined by Cohen & Omery (1994).

Schools of phenomenology

It has been shown thus far that phenomenology is an approach within continental philosophy. For purposes of qualitative research, however, phenomenology has also been adapted and used as a framework within the so-called interpretive tradition which broadly includes grounded theory and ethnography as Lowenberg (1993) points out. She states: 'Basic to all these approaches is the recognition, of the interpretive and constitutive cognitive processes inherent in all social life' (p. 58) and shows that there are many 'quandaries in terminology' which lead to misinterpretations in the nursing and education research literature, and sometimes in social research. She argues that there is a problem with phenomenology, the distinctions between the assumptions that lie behind the theories (e.g. Husserl and Heidegger) and the actual method, the 'doing' of phenomenology. Part of the purpose of this chapter is to try and unravel these perplexities.

The useful outline of phenomenological philosophy guiding research and developing into schools that have different approaches, is presented by Cohen & Omery (1994). However, they do highlight that the broad goal in each school remains the same, that is to gain knowledge about phenomena.

We have developed Fig. 8.1 from the writing of Cohen & Omery (1994). This depicts three schools. According to Cohen & Omery the first is the so-called Duquesne school guided by Husserl's ideas about eidetic structure. The second school is about the interpretation of phenomena (Heideggerian hermeneutics). The combination of both is found in the so-called Dutch school. The Duquesne school focuses mostly on the notion of description. The 'interpretation of phenomena' approach concentrates on taken for granted practices and common meanings, whilst the Dutch school aims to combine both description and interpretation.

It has been argued recently (Streubert & Carpenter, 1995) that phenomenology is, in fact, an integral research approach that involves philosophical, sociological and psychological perspectives. These authors also contend that, whilst it is a useful method for examining phenomena important to nursing (and, we would add, midwifery), it still remains relatively new. In consequence a number of confusions arise. Streubert & Carpenter (1995) suggest that researchers new to phenomenology are often uncertain of how to proceed. The process of phenomenological research will now be outlined, with specific approaches to data analysis.

The phenomenological research process

Van Manen (1990) argues that phenomenological research is primarily about wanting to know the world in which we live. As such the world's *secrets* as he puts it, and *intimacies* that form experience of the world, are questioned and examined. He

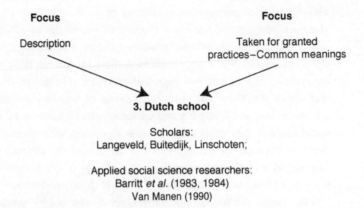

1. Eidetic structure

Guided by Husserl
Duquesne School-Approaches
developed by
researchers:
Giorgi, Colaizzi, Fischer and van Kaam

Focus

Description

2. Interpretation of phenomena

Guided by Heidegger
'Heideggerian Hermeneutics'

Nurse researchers include:
Benner (1984)
Benner and Wrubel (1989)
Diekelmann, Allen and Tanner (1989)

Focus

Taken for granted
practices–Common meanings

3. Dutch school

Scholars:
Langeveld, Buitedijk, Linschoten;

Applied social science researchers:
Barritt *et al.* (1983, 1984)
Van Manen (1990)

Focus

Combination of description and interpretation

Fig. 8.1   Schools of phenomenology for applied research.

argues that wanting to do this research becomes a 'caring act' (Van Manen, 1990:5) and outlines some important points which identify phenomenological research. Oiler Boyd (1993:126–128) summarises these:

(1) Phenomenological research is the study of lived experience.
(2) Phenomenological research is the explication of phenomena as they present themselves to consciousness.
(3) Phenomenological research is the study of essences.
(4) Phenomenological research is the description of the experiential meanings we live as we live them.
(5) Phenomenological research is the human scientific study of phenomena.
(6) Phenomenological research is the attentive practice of thoughtfulness. Oiler Boyd (1993:127) describes this: 'The impetus, for doing research is the researcher's everyday practical concerns in her or his orientation as nurse for example'.
(7) Phenomenological research is a search for what it means to be human.
(8) Phenomenological research is a poetizing activity. Oiler Boyd (1993:128) summarises this: 'phenomenological description is then characterized by inspirational insight won through reflective writing. Research and writing are thus closely related'.

To begin the process of phenomenological enquiry, the researcher obviously needs an area of interest, puzzlement or concern, or a gap in general or specific knowledge about a phenomenon. Streubert & Carpenter (1995) suggest that professional nursing orientation towards holistic care provides the background for deciding whether to undertake phenomenological research. We would argue that 'holistic care involves a multi-dimensional understanding of health (and illness) that is concerned with physical, emotional and spiritual aspects of health' (Wheeler 1995:50). This holistic perspective, coupled with the study of lived experience, provides the foundation for phenomenological research.

Streubert & Carpenter (1995) advise that the researcher should ask several questions about the intended topic. For example: Is there some need for clarity concerning a phenomenon? Has there been anything published in relation to this, or is there a need for further enquiry? If there is, the nurse researcher should question whether enquiry concerning the lived experience is the most appropriate approach to collecting data. As the accounts of those experiencing the phenomenon are the primary data, the researcher needs to consider that this will yield both rich and descriptive data. Streubert & Carpenter advise that researchers examine their own style preference and ability to engage with this approach to research. Further considerations for the research process concern completion and presentation of the study to relevant audiences.

Appropriate areas for this type of research include:

'... those that are central to the life experience of human beings. Examples include feeling happiness or fear, being there, being committed, being a chairperson or head nurse, or the meaning of stress for nursing students in the clinical setting. Health related topics suitable for phenomenological investigation might include the meaning of pain, quality of life with a particular chronic illness or loss of a body part.'

(Streubert and Carpenter, 1995:35).

A 10-year review of the Cumulative Index to Nursing and Allied Health Literature 1983–1993, conducted by Beck (1994), produced 27 published phenomenological research studies (including that of Clarke & Wheeler, 1992). Beck points out that there were few published phenomenological studies in the 1970s, with a large increase in the latter part of the 1980s, and this is continuing in the 1990s. The studies Beck found covered a range of topic areas including caring in nursing practice, caring between nursing students and physically/mentally disabled children, meaningful life experiences of the elderly, women with advanced breast cancer, infertility in couples, post-partum depression, loss of a partner due to AIDS, chronic illness and relationships in health care, addiction, violence and therapeutic touch. These examples illustrate the breadth of phenomenological research and the potential of this method of enquiry.

Clarke (1991) used a phenomenological approach to investigate the meaning of caring from interviews with six staff nurses. In 1994 Lodi interviewed six individuals with a chronic condition and used a phenomenological enquiry to examine the lived experience of multiple sclerosis. In these studies research participants were volunteers and the usual ethical issues were considered carefully. In this and other aspects of the research process, phenomenological research follows the same sequence as other qualitative enquiry.

In all research approaches the researcher has a responsibility to justify the type of theoretical framework (e.g. symbolic interactionism, phenomenology or any other) and specify and outline the approach to data analysis (e.g. grounded theory for the former, or Colaizzi's or other writers' approaches in the latter). Baker *et al.* (1992) argue that there is a need to clearly define the methodology to avoid 'method-slurring' (we develop this further in Chapter 14).

In data analysis for phenomenological enquiry, the researcher aims to uncover and produce a description of the lived experience. The procedural steps to achieve this aim vary with the approach taken by the researcher in terms of the three main types of phenomenology previously outlined. Ray (1994) points out that data analysis in eidetic or descriptive phenomenology requires the researcher to make full use of bracketing (that is to suspend their past experience, knowledge or prediction of phenomena). Intuition and reflection are important in the data analysis process to help open up 'the meaning of experience both as discourse and as text' (Ray 1994:129).

Approaches to data analysis which follow the requirements of bracketing, intuition and reflection have been developed by various researchers (Fig. 8.1, point 1). One of these, Colaizzi (1978), outlined a seven-stage process of analysis. Although there has been criticism of pioneering work such as this (Hycner, 1985), we have found this particular process of analysis (with some modification) for the eidetic approach of phenomenology to be both logical and credible. Yet we would take the view of Hycner (1985:279) that 'there is an appropriate reluctance on the part of phenomenologists to focus too much on specific steps in research methods for fear that they will become verified as they have in the natural sciences'.

There are, however, several interpretations of the data analysis process depending on the school of phenomenology chosen. For example Streubert & Carpenter (1995) outline the different procedural steps from six authors: van Kaam (1959), Paterson & Zderad (1976), Colaizzi (1978), Van Manen (1984), Giorgi (1985) and Streubert (1991).

The 27 phenomenological research studies reviewed by Beck (1994) appeared to be guided by the Duquesne school and used the approaches from one of the following authors: Colaizzi (1978), Giorgi (1985) or van Kaam (1966). In consequence Beck outlines the different procedural steps for data analysis developed by them. Colaizzi advocates seven steps, Giorgi four and van Kaam six.

In selecting a school of phenomenology the researcher will be guided by the approach to the most appropriate procedural steps in data analysis. For the purposes of this chapter, we outline and discuss those developed by Colaizzi (1978). It is, however, a decision for student and supervisor (novice or expert researcher) to select the approach best suited for the phenomenon under investigation and utilise the appropriate literature to guide the research methodology and analysis.

Colaizzi (1978) argues a case for descriptive research and provides a method for data analysis, for instance from transcribed tapes of interviews with participants. Again we would state that this is one approach available to the researcher, there are others.

The seven-stage process of analysis occurs as follows:

(1) The first task of the researcher is to read the participants' narratives to acquire a feeling for their ideas in order to understand them.
(2) The next step involves the researcher in extracting words and sentences relating to the phenomenon under study. Colaizzi calls this process *extracting significant statements*.
(3) The researcher then attempts to *formulate meanings* for each significant statement.
(4) The researcher repeats this process for each description from the participant and arranges these formulated means into *clusters of themes*.
    (a) The researcher returns to the original descriptions to validate the themes.
    (b) At this stage there may be contradictions among or between the groups of themes. The researcher is advised by Colaizzi to resist the temptation to ignore data or themes which do not fit.
(5) Following this step, the researcher is able to integrate all the resulting ideas into an *exhaustive description* of the phenomenon under study.
(6) The researcher then reduces the exhaustive description of the phenomenon to an essential structure. Colaizzi describes this as an *unequivocal statement of identification of the fundamental structure* of the phenomenon.
(7) In the final stage the researcher returns to the participants in the research for a further interview to elicit their views on the findings and to validate them.

These are the descriptions of procedural steps from Colaizzi (1978:59–61).

Colaizzi encourages researchers to be flexible with these stages, and we have found this to be useful. For example, we have encouraged students to take the exhaustive description back to informants, rather than the final, essential structure, because it appears to be more recognisable for them for comment. This ensures rigour (see also Chapter 12).

To illustrate the stages of analysis we will refer to Clarke's (1991) study. The extracts used are small snapshots and therefore, viewed in isolation from the complete study, can only serve to give a basic guide. It is the convention for students to include in the appendix of the study whole interview transcripts or important parts of these and link them with significant statements, formulated meanings and theme clusters to show how the data emerge. The *exhaustive description* and the final *essential structure* are presented in the findings section of the study.

Example

A view of the phenomenon of caring in nursing practice
Each participant's description was taped and transcribed verbatim.

In the true spirit of bracketing (*epoché*) the researcher clearly states her own assumptions and meanings of caring in order to attempt to suspend them.

The initial question that was asked of each informant was: 'as a nurse, what is caring for you?'

Stage 1
Interview transcripts were read through repeatedly to acquire a feeling for them.

Stage 2
One transcript was taken at a time. Through concentrating on the transcript page by page, significant statements were noted from each page pertaining to the 'caring' example below.

PARTICIPANT: 'I think if you want to create a caring image you have to give a lot of yourself, and if I am prepared to give information and am prepared to talk to patients, spend time with them and not begrudge anything I do for the patient, I think that this is caring and I think that they will definitely get the positive vibes from that and feel cared for, feel as if somebody cares.'
INTERVIEWER: 'So it is giving part of you?'
PARTICIPANT: 'I think so. I think it can be really exhausting as well, because all day long you are giving so much of yourself. You are giving all day to your job, otherwise you cannot do it.'

Significant statements:
(1) You have to give a lot of yourself.
(2) Really exhausting as well because all day long, you are giving so much of yourself.

Stage 3
Creative insight, suggested by Colaizzi, was needed at this stage. However, it was important not to formulate meanings which were unconnected to the data. Clarke (1991:45) points out that it is very important to refer back to the original data ... 'to ensure that the original words and meanings of the informants were used'.

Formulated meaning example:
The voluntary giving all day to patients and colleagues is exhausting and leaves little reserves on returning home.

Stage 4
A theme in each formulated meaning was identified and written down as a theme key. The theme key was numbered with the source number of the

Example *contd.*

formulated meaning. This facilitated identification of the theme key to the formulated meaning.

Example of formulated meaning:
13. A caring ability is innate and cultured during primary socialisation.

Theme key
Source of care 5, 13
Groupings started to develop from these theme keys which led to tentative theme clusters. At this stage, it is important to 'continually refer back to formulated meanings, significant statements and the original transcription to ensure the linkages were accurate'. (Clarke 1991:46).

Following this, categories are firmed up using the informants' words where possible as category titles. There were four: caring ability, being supportive, communicating and pressure.

Stage 5
This involves integration of the data into an exhaustive description which again involves 'contemplative dwelling' to construct a description that is true to the data.

Stage 6
The exhaustive description was taken back to participants for verification. They were interviewed again. The nurse researcher used a short interview guide.

Stage 7
This stage requires a further reduction of the exhaustive description into an essential structure of the phenomenon of caring.

Essential structure of caring:
'Care is a continuous process of need, that is experienced through the giving of oneself to another, creating friendship through trust, respect, love and value for each other.

Communication in active and receptive modes is exercised to assist patients, together with the understanding that a physical presence can provide comfort for them. Nurses seek awareness of patients' needs to utilise those skills in physical and psychological areas to promote potential patient independence.

Nurses empathise with patients and relatives to recognise the anxiety and distress that they experience, and, through being supportive, try to alleviate such anxiety.

Caring is rewarding and exhausting. Pressures are experienced from patients, managers, the clinical areas and themselves. These affect the quality

Example *contd.*

of care they can give. Ability to care is reflected in personal receipt of care, instinct and professional knowledge, which all build personal confidence' (Clarke 1991:59).

Summary

Phenomenology is primarily a philosophy within the so-called continental tradition. There are three main phases in the movement (preparatory, German and French) and key figures are Husserl, Heidegger and Sartre. These writers developed different conceptual formulations – very broadly, descriptive (Husserl), interpretive (Heidegger) and ontological-existential (Sartre) – which have been adapted as methods of enquiry by researchers. Authors and researchers have been directed in their approaches by these ideas and form three different schools of phenomenology: eidetic structure (Husserlian), interpretation of phenomena (Heideggerian) and the Dutch school (combination of approaches).

Methods of data analysis have been formulated by researchers in the different schools. The process of research as suggested by one of these, Colaizzi, has been outlined and demonstrated in an example.

References

Baker C., Wuest J. & Stern, P.N. (1992) Method slurring: the grounded theory/phenomenology example. *Journal of Advanced Nursing*, **17**, 1355–1360.

Beck C.T. (1994) Phenomenology: its use in nursing research. *International Journal of Nursing Studies*, **31**(6), 449–510.

Benner P. (1984) *From Novice to Expert: Excellence and Power in Clinical Nursing Practice.* Addison-Wesley, Menlo Park, California.

Benner P. & Wrubel J. (1989) *The Primacy of Caring: Stress and Coping in Health and Illness.* Addison-Wesley, Menlo Park, California.

Bleicher J. (1980) *Contemporary Hermeneutics: Hermeneutics of Method, Philosophy and Critique.* Routledge and Kegan Paul, London.

Clarke J.B. (1991) *A view of the phenomenon of caring in nursing.* Unpublished BSc study, Bournemouth University, Bournemouth.

Clarke J.B. & Wheeler S.J. (1992) A view of the phenomenon of caring in nursing practice. *Journal of Advanced Nursing*, **17**, 1283–1290.

Cohen M.Z. (1987) A historical overview of the phenomenologic movement. *Image: Journal of Nursing Scholarship*, **19**(1), 31–34.

Cohen M. Z. & Omery A. (1994) Schools of phenomenology: implications for research. In *Critical Issues in Qualitative Research Methods* (ed. J.M. Morse), pp. 136–156, Sage, Thousand Oaks, California.

Colaizzi P. (1978) Psychological research as a phenomenologist views it. In *Existential*

Phenomenological Alternatives for Psychology (eds R. Valle & M. King), pp. 48–71, Oxford University Press, New York.

Diekelmann N., Allen D. & Tanner C. (1989) *The NLN Criteria for Appraisal of Baccalaureate Programs: A Critical Hermaneutic Analysis*. National League for Nursing Press, New York.

Heidegger M. (1962) *Being and Time*. Translated by J. Macquarrie & E. Robinson. Harper and Row, New York.

Hycner R.H. (1985) Some guidelines for the phenomenological analysis of interview data. *Human Studies*, 8, 279–303.

Koch T. (1995) Interpretive approaches in nursing research: the influence of Husserl and Heidegger. *Journal of Advanced Nursing*, 21, 827–836.

Leonard V.W. (1994) A Heideggerian phenomenological perspective on the concept of person. In *Interpretive Phenomenology: Embodiment, Caring and Ethics in Health and Illness* (ed. P. Benner), pp. 43–63, Sage, Thousand Oaks, California.

Lodi Y. (1994) The lived experience of multiple sclerosis: a phenomenological inquiry. Unpublished BSc study, Bournemouth University, Bournemouth.

Lowenberg J.S. (1993) Interpretive research methodology: broadening the dialogue. *Advances in Nursing Science*, 16(2), 57–69.

Oiler Boyd C. (1993) Phenomenology: the method. In *Nursing Research: A Qualitative Perspective* (eds P.L. Munhall & C. Oiler Boyd), pp. 99–132, National League for Nursing Press, New York.

Priest S. (1991) *Theories of Mind*. Penguin, Harmondsworth.

Ray M. (1994) The richness of phenomenology: philosophic, theoretic and methodologic concerns. In *Critical Issues in Qualitative Research Methods* (ed. J.M. Morse), pp. 117–135, Sage, Thousand Oaks, California.

Spiegelberg H. (1971) *The Phenomenological Movement: A Historical Introduction* 2nd edn, Volumes 1 & 2, Martinus Nijhoff, The Hague.

Streubert H.J. & Carpenter D.R. (1995) *Qualitative Research in Nursing: Advancing the Human Imperative*. J.B. Lippincott, Philadelphia.

Taylor B.J. (1994) *Being Human: Ordinariness in Nursing*. Churchill Livingstone, Melbourne.

Teichman J. & Evans K.C. (1991) *Philosophy, A Beginner's Guide*. Blackwell Science, Oxford.

The Chambers Dictionary (1993) Chambers Harrop, Edinburgh.

The New Concise Oxford English Dictionary (1993) Clarendon Press, Oxford.

Van Manen M. (1990) *Researching Lived Experience: Human Science for an Action Sensitive Pedagogy*. State Unversity of New York Press, New York.

Vessey G. & Foulkes P. (1990) *Collins Dictionary of Philosophy*. Collins, Glasgow.

Walters A.J. (1955) The phenomenological movement: implications for nursing research. *Journal of Advanced Nursing*, 22, 791–799.

Wheeler S.J. (1995) Child abuse: the health perspective. In *Family Violence and the Caring Professions* (eds P. Kingstone & B. Penhale), pp. 50–76, Macmillan, Basingstoke.

Chapter 9

Feminist Approaches and Qualitative Research

This chapter will describe:

- The origins of feminist methodology in feminist theory
- The methodology
- The problems of feminist methodology

Many feminist studies, though not all, use qualitative data collection and analysis for a variety of reasons. Some feminists believe in a separate and distinctive feminist research methodology, and that this type of enquiry is not merely a variation or branch of qualitative research (Stanley & Wise, 1983, 1993). Harding (1987), however, suggests that a distinctive feminist method does not exist, but that feminist researchers address certain epistemological and methodological issues. Indeed, one might argue that many feminist researchers do not differentiate between methodology and method (King, 1994). We would like to remind researchers that methodology includes the principles and theoretical perspectives underlying research; methods are the strategies or techniques for collecting and analysing data.

Feminist method should rightly be called feminist methodology. The latter gives the research its special character because the overall principles are feminist (Campbell & Bunting, 1991). The guidelines for feminist research relate to attitudes, cognition and emotion rather than presenting strict rules for 'doing' research (Reinharz, 1992). This methodology is concerned with giving women the opportunity to voice their concerns and interests, and not with the technical details of data analysis. The latter depends on the field in which researchers work and on the specific research question.

Methods too, reflect the feminist principles of equality between researcher and participant, and focus on women's experiences and their empowerment; hence feminists use qualitative methods. The favoured type of data collection tends to be life history interviews or narratives, 'letting the women speak'. Taking into account the requirements of feminist research, researchers use grounded theory, ethnography and other types of data analysis. The focus on the *lived experience* means that phenomenological approaches are often taken in nursing research.

Griffin (1995) uses the term which has gained acceptance: feminist standpoint research. It is a less specific term than feminist methodology, which carries with it the implication that feminist research is a specific type of analysis. Feminist standpoint research recognises that the view of the world by feminist researchers is distinctive and different, while the particular strategies of analysis are of lesser importance, although there should be a fit between the world view and the methods adopted.

In this chapter, however, we are not concerned with nomenclature, but with feminist thought about doing research and feminists' actions as researchers. A number of major issues emerge in thinking and doing research within a feminist methodological framework:

(1)   An initial reaction against positivist research and traditional strategies which were seen as male-dominated and androcentric.

(2)   A desire and interest to explore women's perceptions, experiences and feelings; that is to make women visible.

(3)   An emphasis on the feminist principles of equality which changes the relationship between researcher and researched.

(4)   The use of consciousness-raising as a methodological tool to empower women.

(5)   The centrality of feminist theory and the aim to add to this via research.

The origins of feminist methodology

Feminist methodology has its roots in feminist theory. Writers such as Millett (1969), Mitchell (1971) and Oakley (1972), as well as others, particularly in the US and Britain, were the pioneers who helped to direct the focus on women's interests and ideas.

One of the early seminal chapters in Britain on feminist research was written by Oakley (1981). It created an awareness of the importance of relationships in interviewing which has become one of the central issues in feminist research. In nursing in Britain the discussion started with an article by Webb (1984).

More recently a number of books by Stanley & Wise (1983, 1993) and Fonow & Cook (1991a) have contained chapters specifically concerning feminist research methodology and techniques, while the book by Reinharz (1992) is wholly concerned with feminist methodology and techniques.

Feminist theory

Feminist theory and method are so closely interwoven that they cannot be fully separated, and therefore a discussion of theory is necessary. Feminist methodology has its basis in feminist theories, complex and multi-stranded constructions about women's perspectives, oppression and consciousness. Feminist theory is an exploration of the values of feminism. Stanley & Wise (1983) trace the emergence of feminist theory to the 1960s and 1970s, when writers (such as those above) discussed women's oppression, exploitation and inequalities. They saw this oppression mainly as structural, that is, built into the structure of society and institutions as well as emerging from patterns of socialisation.

Stanley & Wise (1993) argue that it is impossible to speak of feminist theory as though it were a single entity. Theory initially developed on a macro-level, involving society, institutions and patterns of power. The micro-level, related to individuals and their interaction with each other, was also examined. The latter is more important for nurse researchers who deal with interactions between individuals such as colleagues and patients/clients. Early feminist theories developed from an emphasis on the description and critique of positivism. Later feminists stress personal action and experience.

Feminist theories in the words of Stanley & Wise (1993) are 'a set of theoretical constructions' about women's oppression and the way that this oppression is linked to the nature of social reality. Some of the tenets of feminism, such as a belief in the oppression of women, are shared by most feminists. They work to uncover the cultural bias in favour of men and to undermine the system which oppresses women. Sartori (1994), however, when talking about women in science, argues that women's lack of authority may be the problem rather than male oppression.

Denny (1994) debates one of the paradoxes and difficulties of radical feminism, which, she claims, might lead to an oppression of women, the very thing feminists try to prevent. Denny gives as an example feminists who suggest that reproductive technologies are controlled by men, and that women are not even aware of this. While there may be an element of truth in this assertion, Denny believes that not all women with experience of reproductive technology are passive and unaware of controls. Her own research (Denny 1994) on *in-vitro* fertilisation showed that, on the contrary, women were aware of limits to their choices and are not merely passive recipients of others' decisions.

Methodology

Feminist researchers emphasise an alternative social reality and value women's lives and experience. These writers seek to make people aware that patriarchy is embedded in social relationships, and they try to demonstrate the lack of mystique in the belief about the 'naturalness of patriarchal relations' (Cook & Fonow, 1986). These relations are not only embedded in the structure of society but have taken part in the construction of social relationships.

Researchers intend to contribute to the improvement of the lives of women. The radical tenet of feminist methods is concerned with the importance of women's lives, and their position in the social structure; 'feminists are interested in women as individuals and as a social category' (Reinharz, 1992:241).

For nurses and midwives this is of particular importance, as most of them are women and can adopt a woman's perspective. Nursing, a profession that is overwhelmingly female, has relatively low status. Feminist research in nursing addresses some of these issues and makes women more visible. Seibold *et al.* (1994) claim that feminist research implies that the principal researcher is a woman. Empathy with women may be easier to achieve by female researchers because of their gender (though feminists do not claim that men cannot have empathy, nor that research supports a woman's perspective just because it is done by a woman).

Fonow & Cook (1991b) assert that feminist research emphasises the affective elements in research with human beings which can provide insight into social reality. The relationship to nursing is clearly established here. Women in our society have been socialised into caring roles and and are committed to the welfare of the research participants (Gilligan, 1982). Through their upbringing, they are more familiar with sharing and expressing their emotions.

The critique of the 'objective' natural science approach

Even before feminism, a disenchantment with natural scientific methods had emerged which led to a critique of the positivist paradigm (as discussed in Chapter 1) which had its roots in the ideas of the philosopher Comte. His model of the social sciences adopted the tenets of natural science, namely the belief that social life is ruled by natural laws which must be found through scientific methods in a similar way to that in biology or physics. Researchers who took the approach of natural science believed that objectivity was possible and that to use the scientific method was the best way to examine social reality. They thought that social reality could be uncovered through 'unbiased' measurement and observation and therefore be value-free and impersonal (DePoy & Gitlin, 1993). Feminists question the whole idea of a value-neutral science in social research (Stanley & Wise, 1983, Stanley 1990). In this they agree with other qualitative researchers who react against this traditional positivist research.

Feminist critics of this approach maintain that it is often stripped of its context while questions and answers are predefined and controlled by researchers who, whilst claiming objectivity, impose their own subjective framework. The tenets of positivism were based on the belief in an objective and universal truth and the 'science' of a quantitative analytical method to uncover this. Gorelick (1991) suggests that the claim of value-free and objective science is 'pretence' and 'presumption'. Feminists believe that researchers cannot achieve complete objectivity. All they can do is state their biases and demonstrate the value bases from which they come. This does not mean that quantitative methods are never adopted, and indeed they are sometimes defended.

Feminists call the traditional research styles 'male-stream' (mainstream) social science for a variety of reasons. They neglected women's experiences and ideas. The personal experience of women was denied validity. Women are treated as inferior, and this fact has implications for the whole of society and not just for women. Feminists claim that personal experience is real and valid. They criticise the differentiation between the objective and subjective and put an emphasis on the relationships and realities of everyday life, through which social structures can be understood. Reinharz (1992) asserts that the subjectivity/objectivity debate becomes obsolete. The social reality of women is demonstrated in personal accounts which women give of their lives, and these accounts emerge from their shared experiences. The researcher listens to these accounts and, while interpreting them, gives a faithful picture of the personal histories and biographies of women.

The relationship between researcher and researched

In feminist enquiry the research relationship between the investigator and the participant differs from that of traditional methods. A number of feminist researchers criticise this view of the relationship that researchers have with the participants in their study. Early researchers had taken, or so feminists believe, a 'spectator attitude' (Stanley & Wise, 1983; Mies, 1991; Gorelick, 1991) which meant that they detached themselves from the people they interviewed or observed and looked at them in a supposedly neutral and objective way.

Traditional research texts advised social scientists to create rapport in the hope that this would generate more and better data; a practical and pragmatic view, although occasionally they warned against over-rapport, fearing that this might damage objectivity. Researchers detached themselves from the participants in their enquiry, who were seen as passive subjects whose views could be examined from the outside. In fact, feminists see this detached relationship as one of exploitation.

Oakley (1981), in her now famous article on women's experiences of talking to researchers, particularly points to the importance of the research relationship in interviewing. She criticises impersonal relationships between interviewer and the person interviewed, because they result in an interview which becomes a mechanistic tool for data collection. It transforms the participants – active human beings – into passive recipients of the researcher's questions and mere respondents. On the other hand, Oakley points out that some of the advice for so-called non-directive interviews which allow free range thought might be flawed because the interviewer uses the procedures of psychoanalysis. Both types of interview involve hierarchy, emotional detachment and the dominance of one group of people over another, rather than a reciprocal relationship between researcher and researched.

The link between researcher and researched in feminist research is very strong, and the interaction between them becomes an integral part of the research. Women must be allowed, even encouraged, to ask questions of the researcher to emphasise reciprocity, so that the research can become a joint enterprise. The life experiences that researched and researchers share can bring them closer together, enhance the relationship and advance knowledge about women for women. In 1984 Webb wrote her classic article 'Feminist methodology in nursing research'. In this she argues strongly that the subjectivity of the researcher and the interests of the participants should be taken into account.

Example

Webb (1984) discusses research which she undertook with a group of women undergoing hysterectomies for non-cancerous conditions (Webb, 1983). She organised two study groups, one group to be interviewed 3 to 4 weeks prior to surgery and 3 months post-surgery. The other group was to be interviewed only once at 3 months post-surgery.

Example *contd.*

In the first group, Webb found that, even while she was arranging the pre-surgery interview, women asked on the phone if she would answer questions when she visited. During the interviews the first study group had many questions and criticisms concerning the management of their impending surgery.

Webb felt that she did not want to exploit the women and wished to give something in return for the rich data she obtained. Therefore she told them to see the interview as an 'exchange of information'. She not only answered questions but gave information and advice when a need for it arose.

Webb sees the sharing of experiences as an important aspect of feminist research and includes in her study (described above) a discussion of involvement with participants through her own experience as a patient. This aspect of involvement is one of the reasons why many feminists advise that women should only be resear-ched by other women in an easy informal manner which establishes a non-hier-archical relationship (Finch, 1984). Being of the same gender and sharing experiences with the researcher generates a feeling of trust and a willingness to communicate ideas. Researcher and informant approach a position of equality. The researcher is not only seen as an expert scholar or academic but as a human being with her own experiences, and this gives her access to other women's feelings and thoughts.

Reinharz (1992) points out that there are no strict distinctions between the formal relationship of the researcher and participant and personal links between them. Sometimes informants and researchers even become friends and form a lasting link. Feminists suggest that the participants should have a choice in the topic area and direction of the research as well as becoming involved in the analysis. This means that the relations between researcher and researched are non-hierarchical; the researcher does not impose control or a power relationship. In nursing this is not easy. As we mentioned before, the very relationship between the professional with expertise and specialist skills, and the clients who are not always knowl-edgeable about their condition, may involve an imbalance of power.

For these reasons the personal experience and values of the researcher become important in feminist research. Feminists often describe and integrate their own feelings while recounting and analysing women's experiences, pains and passions. Often they study women's conditions or problems that they have experienced in their own lives. Reinharz (1992) states that female researchers start with a research question linked to their own experience, often adopting a woman's perspective. A nurse with breast cancer may decide to collect data from women with breast cancer, or a midwife who has had a miscarriage might study women with the same experience. Of course, having an illness or a problem should not be a requirement to researching it.

Although a personal problem or question makes the health professional more aware and sensitive to other women's feelings, it would be dangerous to automatically transfer one's own feelings and thoughts to those of others. Overidentification could generate assumptions and prevent careful listening to the accounts of women, although self-disclosure of the interviewer can help participants to verbalise their own feelings. An exchange of information can be valuable.

Example

Wilde (1992), in examining critical factors influencing nurses' perceptions of their performance in specific situations, found that she needed to break the conventional rules of not being involved in the research interview. So strong was the dilemma of not wanting to detract from the interviews yet 'wanting to support the participants in their sharing of sensitive material', that she produced a paper to examine this tension and analyse the relationship between researcher and informant.

Wilde argues that the nurse as researcher cannot ignore all her other roles when interacting with participants and adds that researchers have the obligation to help the participants gain meaning from their experience. This is not a negative influence on the research but enhances it; the nurse has to respond to the participant as a person which produces beneficial effects for both. In Wilde's view it is impossible for a qualitative researcher to have a detached relationship with the informant.

Valuing others, adopting a position of equality towards the clients and empathising with them while seeing them as human beings and not numbers are, in any case, the principles that are inherent in the caring professions and qualitative research. Indeed, Webb (1984, 1993) believes that adopting a 'sharing, non-hierarchical approach' with patients would improve nursing care because this approach enhances the understanding of their emotions and needs. Reinharz (1983) even advises that informants should take part in the data analysis, identifying major issues of concern, as this helps them to focus on areas which are important to them.

Feminist qualitative research allows for interactive interviewing where participants can ask questions, both professional and personal. In nursing research with patients this becomes important. Patients who can ask questions and engage in a conversation do not feel exploited. If the researcher does not have the answer, she can help the informant to find somebody with the expertise to answer them.

Cook & Fonow (1986) argue that this type of research avoids the objectification of the participant and rejects earlier beliefs that a strict separation between researcher and research 'subject' makes the study more objective. In feminist research different relationships should be developed. Female researchers have 'double vision', because on the one hand, they can see the world from a woman's perspective, and on the other they are scholars and academics who are involved in a piece of scientific research. The interactive methods which take equality as a baseline create awareness in the interviewee of her own power and possibilities because she develops confidence in this situation.

In order to arrive at descriptions of lived experiences, interaction between the researcher and the participant will need to occur in the in-depth interview. How can the researchers establish a relationship of equality when they impose a framework on the participants and give questionnaires to them which direct their answers? Because of these problems there is a stronger relationship between feminist research and qualitative methods. Both feminist and qualitative research stress the importance of a close researcher–researched relationship.

There is an essential tension, and sometimes even a conflict, between the research relationship and the attempt to achieve the research goal of generating information. Acker *et al.* (1991) warn of possible exploitation of the friendship and closeness between researcher and participant which might be used to manipulate the informants. Beck (1994) highlights the problems in phenomenology of the use of self. The self is the main research instrument in qualitative research. Beck asks questions about using the self while at the same time bracketing it out: there is always a conflict for the researcher who needs to be both involved in the study and yet out of it (Lipson et al., 1991). The aims of the enquirer and the informant are never wholly congruous regardless of the position of power which is occupied by the two parties in the the the research. Stanley & Wise (1993:63) speak of 'the essential validity of personal experience'. Stanley (1994) develops the writing of self as 'narratives, lives and autobiography'. She argues for not excising the self from these writings because it is complex and interrelated to other selves.

A critique of male domination and androcentricity

In the past, forms of enquiry were often designed by men and from a male perspective. Traditional research is described by feminists as male dominated (Westkott, 1990) for a variety of reasons:

- It is hierarchical
- It aims for detachment and unachievable objectivity
- It exploits participants

This type of research fails to make explicit the construction and knowledge production in research dominated by male researchers, who see the data and the participants from the male point of view and therefore might distort both the data and the experiences of the informants.

Feminists claim that the social and political context of our society creates bias towards the male point of view. Not only do men occupy a position of power but our very language and conceptualisation lead many researchers, even women, to adopt a male perspective on the world and hence on research design, methods and data. This androcentricity ignores the influence of gender. The resulting ideas and theories often pertain to one gender only but claim generality and applicability to both (this happens particularly in historical research).

Example

An example in health research could be given: in a study of interaction between nurses and patients, the gender of either group might be completely ignored. In research on the link between unemployment and health, the enquiry might focus on male health only. Researchers often fail to make the omission explicit (whether deliberate or not). It is interesting in this context that in certain occupations women are almost entirely ignored.

Terms and language often give the impression of general statements which involve both genders, but many pertain actually to the male gender only. Rarely does this type of research address the concerns of men and women; indeed, it ignores the significance of gender (Eichler, 1988) and might lead researchers to take the male gender as the norm. In the health professions the gender of the researcher is of particular importance. Women's conditions are often researched by male researchers who have never had and will never have these experiences.

Example of research from the women's perspective

Seibold *et al.* (1994) cite the menopause as an example. The writers claim that this has been investigated by male doctors in the past. This means that the voices of those with direct access to this female experience cannot be heard. Seibold wished to redress the balance by reporting about the menopause from the women's perspective. She interviewed 20 single women in midlife about their menopausal experiences.

This example had many of the characteristics which feminists demand of feminist research: the topic focused on the experience of women; the researcher was female; and the sample was recruited through networking which gave the women more control.

Feminist researchers suggest that the past dominance of masculinity is shown in four particular areas (Lennon & Whitford, 1994):

- Problems were discussed in terms of male experience
- The structure of masculine gender identity was reflected in theoretical perspectives.
- The interests of men were promoted and those of women subordinated
- Women were seen as beings that lacked masculinity, and the social order favoured men.

Consciousness raising

Feminist research aims to raise the consciousness of people in general and of the women participants in the enquiry specifically. The idea of consciousness-raising initially stems from Freire's ideas (1970), stating that those who are powerless become aware of their lack of power and plan their own actions for change. The basic premises of feminist research include the oppression and powerlessness of women (Scott, 1985).

Researchers try to use consciousness-raising as a tool for narrowing the distance between researchers and participants by generating reciprocity and collaboration. This affects all participants and gives individuals, including researchers, a sense of their identity. Women, so feminists believe, see themselves differently and take new approaches in their lives after becoming aware of their position through the research process and relationships, and they aim to change their situation and actions. Purposeful action will create power for participants. Changed consciousness can change meanings, interpretations and actions. The research act focuses on women and their experiences.

The researcher herself is a member of a group which is weaker personally and professionally than men and can empathise with her informants. Consciousness of their reality can guide women to an understanding and helps them to change their lives. That which was assumed to be 'natural', for instance the dominant position of males, can be questioned and even rejected.

The focus on women's experience

Feminist research explores experiences and issues that generate changes in perception of actions and conditions such as rape, abuse and violence, as well as ordinary domestic situations and the routine elements of women's lives, aspects which differ from those in the lives of men. It makes emotions, personal values and the thoughts of participants legitimate topics of research. Nurse researchers listen to the voices of the informants, and the women themselves show what it feels like being a woman and the problems and joys inherent in their conditions.

Example

A study of women with a history of drinking aimed to examine women's experiences of drinking problems. Using life history data collection, the researcher found out from her informants about negative professional attitudes towards women. Male professionals in particular assumed that women were more difficult to treat, and that their difficulties stemmed from neuroses and personality problems. The women themselves felt stigmatised. The research tried to redress these judgmental attitudes by taking account of the women's own perspectives and thereby empowering them.

(Davison, in preparation)

The most frequent form of data collection is therefore the personal narrative or life history. Women's diverse experiences within the context of their lives become the focus of research. Researchers gain a picture of the whole of women's experiences through their accounts rather than perceiving a fragmented image. The use of narrative is valuable in understanding feminist ontology which is about the theory of being. All qualitative researchers seek to explore, examine, uncover and share the 'lived experience', but, as Hammersley (1995:55) points out, 'they would not usually advocate commitment to a particular group', nor would they actively intervene on behalf of that group.

The debate highlights some of the principles underlying feminist research, which Wuest (1995) summarises as:

- The knowledge generated should be of use to the people studied
- The research methods should not oppress the participants
- The methods should be reflexive

The problems of feminist methodology

The critique of feminist research is concerned with issues such as:

- The importance of gender and the question of exclusivity
- The degree of participant involvement in choice of topic and data analysis
- The problem of relativism

One of the critics of feminist methodology is Hammersley (1992), who, nevertheless, acknowledges the importance of research about gender and deplores the neglect of this topic in past research. He cites Alcoff's (1988) advice that the issue of gender should not have priority over other variables of equal importance. It is questioned whether researchers who adopt a particular stance and claim superior and unique insight into a group by virtue of their own membership of that group and their own experiences, are following a sound methodological path.

The claim that 'differing states of consciousness lead us to constructing different social worlds' (Stanley & Wise, 1983) is seen by Hammersley (1992) as relativism. The emphasis on the uniqueness of women's experiences ignores the social context which involves more than one gender. One might ask the practical question whether a female researcher can ever interview males, or male researchers interview females. If the answer is no, could one not take this further by suggesting that middle-aged researchers must not interview young people, middle class researchers should never research working class participants, and so on.

While it would be useful to have a researcher with a similar gender, background, religion or colour as the participant, this is not always practically possible, nor desirable in all cases. Nevertheless, although feminist research stipulates that the researcher should be a woman, it does not claim that this type of research is the only valid research method. Gender is seen as an intrinsic and valuable connection, but even women are not a homogeneous group (Lennon & Whitford, 1994).

Critics of feminist methods claim that the ideas of feminists are congruent or at least overlap with the main principles of qualitative research and are thus not unique to feminism. The term methodology, says Hammersley (1992), cannot be justified unless it has unique and specific rules and principles. Feminist research, however, uses the data collection and analysis of other methods although it has a distinct basis in feminist theory and epistemology.

Summary

Feminist approaches do not prescribe methods of analysing research but suggest ways of thinking about it. Feminists criticise the androcentric nature of much research; they intend to make women visible, raise their consciousness and empower them. The most common form of feminist research is the narrative or life history, because it gives women the chance to tell their own stories in their own way.

The stance of the researchers is of importance; they recognise that research is not neutral and value-free, and that their subjectivity can become part of their research. The research relationship is one of equality and mutual trust.

Critics of feminist research claim that it is relativist and ignores the social context which involves more than one gender, and that it takes a restricted perspective on social science data.

References

Acker J., Barry K. & Esseveld J. (1991) Objectivity and truth: problems in doing feminist research. In *Beyond Methodology: Feminist Scholarship as Lived Research* (eds M.M. Fonow & J.A. Cook), pp. 133–153, Indiana University Press, Bloomington.

Alcoff L. (1988) Cultural feminism versus post-structuralism: the identity crisis in feminism. *Signs*, 13(3), 405–436.

Beck C. T. (1994) Phenomenology: its use in nursing research. *International Journal of Nursing Studies*, 31(6), 499–510.

Campbell J. & Bunting S. (1991) Voices and paradigms: perspectives and feminist theory. *Advances in Nursing Science*, 13(3), 1–15.

Cook J. A. & Fonow M.M. (1986) Knowledge of women's interests. *Sociological Inquiry*, 56, 2–29.

Davison J. (In preparation) Women with drinking problems. Unfinished PhD study, Southampton University, Southampton.

Denny E. (1994) Liberation or oppression? Radical feminism and in-vitro fertilisation. *Sociology of Health and Illness*, 16(1), 62–79.

DePoy E. & Gitlin L.N. (1993) *Introduction to Research: Multiple Strategies for Health and Human Services*. Mosby, St Louis.

Eichler M. (1988) *Nonsexist Research Methods: A Practical Guide*. Routledge, London.

Finch J. (1984) It's great to have someone to talk to. In *Social Researching: Politics, Problems and Practice* (eds C. Bell & H. Roberts), pp. 70–87, Routledge & Kegan Paul, London.

Fonow M.M. & Cook J.A. (1991a) *Beyond Methodology: Feminist Scholarship as Lived Research*. Indiana University Press, Bloomington.

Fonow M.M. & Cook J.A. (1991b) Back to the future: a look at the second wave of feminist epistemology and methodology. In *Beyond Methodology: Feminist Scholarship as Lived*

Research (eds M.M. Fonow & J.A. Cook), pp. 1–15, Indiana University Press, Bloomington.

Freire P. (1970) *Pedagogy of the Oppressed.* Seabury Press, New York.

Gilligan C. (1982) *In a Different Voice.* Harvard University Press, Cambridge, Massachusetts.

Gorelick S. (1991) Contradictions of feminist methodology. *Gender and Society*, **5**(4), 459–477.

Griffin C. (1995) Feminism, social psychology and qualitative research. *The Psychologist*, **8**(3), 119–121.

Hammersley M. (1992) On feminist methodology. *Sociology*, **26**(2), 187–206.

Hammersley M. (1995) *The Politics of Social Research.* Sage, London.

Harding S. (1987) Introduction. In *Feminism and Methodology* (ed. S. Harding), pp. 1–14, Indiana Press, Bloomington.

King K.E. (1994) Method and methodology in feminist research: what is the difference. *Journal of Advanced Nursing*, **20**, 19–22.

Lennon K. & Whitford M. (1994) Introduction. In *Knowing the Difference: Feminist Perspectives in Epistemology* (eds K. Lennon & M. Whitford), pp. 1–9, Routledge, London.

Lipson J. *et al.* (1991) On bracketing. In *Qualitative Nursing Research: A Contemporary Dialogue* (ed. J.M. Morse), p. 24, Sage, Newbury Park, California.

Mies M. (1991) Women's research or feminist research? The debate surrounding feminist science and methodology. In *Beyond Methodology: Feminist Scholarship as Lived Research* (eds M.M. Fonow & J.A. Cook), pp. 60–84, Indiana University Press, Bloomington.

Millett K. (1969) *Sexual Politics.* Abacus, London.

Mitchell J. (1971) *Women's Estate.* Penguin, Harmondsworth.

Oakley A. (1972) *Sex, Gender and Society.* Temple Smith, London.

Oakley A. (1981) Interviewing women: a contradiction in terms. In *Doing Feminist Research* (ed. H. Roberts), pp. 30–61, Routledge and Kegan Paul, London.

Reinharz S. (1983) Experiential analysis: a contribution to feminist research. In *Theories of Women's Studies* (eds G. Bowles & R. Duelli Klein), pp. 162–191, Routledge and Kegan Paul, London.

Reinharz S. (1992) *Feminist Methods in Social Research.* Oxford University Press, New York.

Sartori D. (1994) Women's authority in science. In *Knowing the Difference: Feminist Perspectives in Epistemology* (eds K. Lennon & M. Whitford), pp. 110–121, Routledge, London.

Scott S. (1985) Feminist research and qualitative methods: a discussion of some of the issues. In *Issues in Educational Research* (ed. R.G. Burgess), pp. 67–85, The Falmer Press, London.

Seibold C., Richards L. & Simon D. (1994) Feminist method and qualitative research about midlife. *Journal of Advanced Nursing*, **19**, 394–402.

Stanley L. (1990) *Feminist Praxis.* Routledge, London.

Stanley L. (1994) The knowing subject: narratives and autobiography. In *Knowing the Difference: Feminist Perspectives in Epistemology* (eds K. Lennon & M. Whitford), pp. 132–148, Routledge, London.

Stanley L. & Wise S. (1983) *Breaking out: Feminist Consciousness and Feminist Research.* Routledge and Kegan Paul, London.

Stanley L. & Wise S. (1993) *Breaking Out Again.* Routledge, London.

Webb C. (1983) Coping with hysterectomy. *Journal of Advanced Nursing*, **8**, 311–319.

Webb C. (1984) Feminist methodology in nursing research. *Journal of Advanced Nursing*, **9**, 249–256.

Webb C. (1993) Feminist research: definitions, methodology, methods and evaluation. *Journal of Advanced Nursing*, **18**, 416–423.

Westkott M. (1990) Feminist criticism of the social sciences. In *Feminist Research Methods. Exemplary Readings in the Social Sciences* (ed. J.M. Nielsen), pp. 58–68, Westview Press, London.

Wilde V. (1992) Controversial hypotheses on the relationship between researcher and informant in qualitative research. *Journal of Advanced Nursing*, **17**, 234–242.

Wuest J. (1995) Feminist grounded theory: an exploration of the congruency and tensions between two traditions in knowledge discovery. *Qualitative Health Research*, **5**(1), 125–137.

In this chapter we shall examine:

- The origin and purpose of focus groups
- The sample size and composition
- How to conduct focus groups
- The involvement of the interviewer
- The analysis of interviews
- Strengths and limitations of focus groups

A focus group involves a number of people with common experiences or characteristics who are interviewed by a researcher (or moderator) for the purpose of eliciting ideas, thoughts and perceptions about a specific topic or certain issues linked to an area of interest.

In the past researchers have used these techniques particularly in the area of marketing and business research, but lately they have become popular in social science and the caring professions. The ideas generated are normally analysed by qualitative methods, although focus groups can result in quantitative or multi-method research. The type of group and the number of interviews is determined by the research question (this is discussed later).

The origin and purpose of focus groups

The first book on focus groups was written by Merton & Kendall in 1946 as a result of working with groups during and shortly after the second world war. This type of in-depth group interview had been used by business and market researchers since the 1920s. It became especially popular in market research in order to gather information about customers' thoughts and feelings about a product, which were seen as important because researchers realised that listening does not only help to improve a product but also stimulates business. If firms take clients' opinions into account, they can provide a product that will be bought.

Today the focus group interview is used by a wide variety of researchers in the areas of communications, policy, marketing and advertising. (Examples of focus groups in market research and their practical uses can be found in the book by Greenbaum, 1988) Only in the last few years has this method of data collection become popular in the caring professions, including nursing, where it is seen as a useful strategy for the evaluation of services, interventions or programmes (Kingry *et al*, 1990). This approach may not be better than other forms of enquiry but it does not rely merely on the initial ideas of the researcher and a single participant; instead, the members of the group generate new questions and ideas. Through these group interviews, professionals are able to discover the needs and feelings of their clients, and the perceptions and attitudes of their colleagues, and they can examine the thoughts of decision makers. Focus groups in the social sciences and health professions have become fashionable since the growth of qualitative research methods in the last 10 or 20 years.

These interviews produce thoughts and opinions about a topic relevant to health care, treatment evaluation and illness experiences.

Example

Morgan & Spanish (1985) for instance, used focus group discussion to demonstrate the impact of social interaction on patients' health belief schemata for heart attacks. The researchers collected tape-recorded group discussions of nine focus groups with 40 participants overall.

Focus groups are characterised by the use of interaction between the participants, from which researchers discover how individuals think and feel about particular issues.

Members of a focus group respond to the interviewer and to each other. The questions might start with eliciting knowledge about a specific condition, the use of a drug or method of intervention to put the members at ease, but should soon go on to a discussion of feelings or thoughts. Different reactions stimulate debate about the topic because group members respond to each other. Discussions in groups might not only develop ideas, problems and questions which researchers have not thought about before, but also find answers to some of these questions.

Patton (1990) stresses that focus groups are not decision making bodies, members need not agree and come to firm and final conclusions. The ultimate goal for the researcher is to understand the reality of the participants, not to make decisions about a specific issue or problem, although future actions may be based on the findings of the focus group interviews.

Focus group interviews differ from interviews with individuals in that they explore and stimulate ideas based on shared perceptions of the world.

The sample: size and composition

The sample is linked closely to the research topic. The people who are interviewed in a focus group usually have similar roles or experiences. They may be colleagues who share the same speciality, or use the same technical equipment or nursing procedures.

Example

One of our colleagues conducted focus group interviews with nurses who had experience of caring for patients who controlled their own pain post-operatively through a device which administers a dose of analgesia intravenously (patient controlled analgesia or PCA). The aim of the study was an exploration of the interaction between patient and nurse and their relationship in this situation. The researcher chose a homogeneous group of 15 registered nurses who were female and aged between 27 and 40 years. She conducted five focus groups consisting of three participants each over a period of two months.

(Ratcliffe, 1994)

Patients in focus groups have undergone common experiences, have the same condition or receive the same treatment. For instance, if a nurse wishes to interview a group of people with diabetes, she or he obviously involves individuals with this condition in the focus groups. Colleagues who are interviewed, generally share common interests, work in similar settings, or perform similar tasks. If the interviewer wants the thoughts of colleagues from a psychiatric setting, for example, then the sample has to be composed of nurses with psychiatric experience. Health promotion, too, is a topic for research, particularly with client groups who are vulnerable or suffer from a specific condition.

Example

Nyamati & Shuler (1990) interviewed groups of black women in the US who were at risk from HIV infection as part of a larger project based on the need to provide a health education programme.

Carey (1994:229) states that the selection of participants generally proceeds 'on the basis of their common experience related to the research topic'. Although group members share experiences, this does not mean that they all have the same views about the topic area, nor that they come from the same background or organisation. It might be useful to recruit members from naturally occurring groups such as antenatal classes or patient support groups. While they have experienced the same conditions, illnesses or events, they are nevertheless heterogeneous in other ways, and so could illuminate the topic from all sides.

The number of focus groups depends on the needs of the researcher and the demands of the topic area. For one research project the usual number is about three or four, but the actual number depends on the complexity of the research topic. The findings from the focus group interviews are often used as a basis for action. A small sample can generate rich data and a great deal of information.

Example

Dignan *et al.* (1990) used a series of four focus groups to examine knowledge and attitudes about cancer screening among black women in an area of the United States. The results of the focus groups interviews showed that the women had little knowledge about the value of early cancer detection and the part that screening took in it. On the basis of the findings health care professionals were able to develop a programme of health education and to use social marketing strategies for making it acceptable.

Studies with large focus groups and many informants exist too. For instance, Hart & Rotem (1990) used 15 groups which included a total of 104 nurses from 44 wards. The normal group involved seven participants. Like other qualitative interviews, group sessions generally last from 1 to 3 hours. We must stress, however, that 3-hour interviews with patients would be far too long and demanding. In market research, participants are paid for their time and effort but not in nursing research, because this would coerce the informants and squander resources. Most new information emerges in the first groups (Kingry *et al.*, 1990); as in other qualitative research important themes often emerge at an early stage.

Each group contains between four and twelve people, but six is probably the optimum number as it is large enough to provide a variety of perspectives and small enough not to become disorderly or fragmented. Indeed, one of our colleagues found that in her experience, a group of six was too large and that the optimum number of members in the group was three. Greenbaum (1988), a writer about market research, however, claims that group dynamics work better if the group is not too small. Slight over-recruitment for each group is advised by Stewart & Shamdasani (1990), two social science researchers, in case of absence of some individuals.

The larger the group, the more difficult the transcription becomes. When several people start talking together and the group becomes lively, it can be difficult to distinguish voices. There may well be a difference between groups who come together for market research purposes and those who gather for health research. The former would feel much less vulnerable because the area of discussion is rarely threatening or sensitive.

Members of the group, although sharing common experiences, do not have to know each other. In a group of immediate colleagues or friends, private thoughts or ideas might not be revealed, although occasionally the opposite could be true. One individual is more likely to dominate others and the past history of the group may inhibit or lead individuals in a particular direction. In nursing research, familiarity between participants, or participants and researcher, could be useful because the 'warm-up' time, the time where informants get to know each other to facilitate interaction, is shorter, and the researcher can focus on the topic immediately. It is believed (Stewart & Shamdasani, 1990) that compatibility among group members is more productive than conflict or hostility, although this too depends on the topic. Sometimes, conflict can generate new and different ideas.

Gender and age of the group members affect the quality and level of interaction and through this the data. For instance, evidence shows greater diversity of ideas in single sex groups than in those of mixed sex (Stewart & Shamdasani, 1990). The latter tend to be more conforming because of the social interaction between males and females; both groups sometimes tend to 'perform' for each other. Krueger (1994) points out that children give natural and spontaneous answers to questions since they find it difficult to pretend, and that they share their feelings more readily. Of course, the topic or the purpose of the focus group generally determines its composition.

Conducting focus group interviews

Focus group interviews must be planned carefully. The informants are contacted well in advance of the interviews and reminded a few days before they start. As in other types of enquiry, ethical and access issues are considered. The environment for a focus group is important as the room must be big enough to contain the participants and the tape recorder needs to be placed in an advantageous location, where they can all be heard and recorded. For focus group work, it is even more essential to have a top quality tape recorder than for individual interviews. Merton & King (1990) suggest a spatial arrangement of a circle or semi-circle, and this seems to be the most successful seating arrangement.

The group interviews should have a clearly identified agenda otherwise they deteriorate into vague and chaotic discussions (Stewart & Shamdasani, 1990). Morgan (1988) believes in the importance of time management because both interviewer and informants have limited time.

From the beginning the researcher establishes ground rules, so that all group members know how to proceed. Researchers plan initial questions and prompts. When the interviews start, the interviewer puts the group at ease and introduces the topic to be debated. Strategies such as showing a film or telling a story related to the topic, sometimes stimulate interaction. Most often questions are asked, and researchers generally proceed from the more general to the specific, just as in other qualitative interviews. Involving all the participants, rather than letting a few individuals dominate the situation demands diplomacy from the researcher, and should be easier with a smaller group. Extreme views in a group of people are balanced out by the reactions of the majority when debating questions.

Focus groups can be combined with individual interviews, observation or other methods of data collection. Morgan & Krueger (1993) maintain that it is not necessary to validate focus interviews by other methods.

The involvement of the interviewer

The interviewer becomes the facilitator or moderator in the group discussion. In nursing or midwifery research, the health professional is the interviewer (while in market research focus groups professional moderators are employed). In health research generally a single interviewer facilitates the groups. Researchers should have the particular qualities of the in-depth interviewer: flexibility, open-mindedness and skill in eliciting information. The creation of an open and non-threatening group climate is one of their initial important tasks. They must be able to stimulate discussion and have insight and interest in the ideas of the informants.

The leadership role of the moderators demands abilities above that of the one-to-one interviewer. They must have the social and refereeing skills to guide the members towards effective interaction and sometimes be able to exert control over informants and topic without directing the debate or coercing the participants. If the group feels at ease with the interviewer, the interaction will be open and productive, and the participants will be comfortable about disclosing their perceptions and feelings.

Morgan (1988) advises that the interviewers hold back on questioning if they want to examine the real feelings of participants; much of the discussion evolves from the dynamics of group interaction. This non-directive approach has particular importance in exploratory research where perceptions are examined. High involvement of the interviewer leads more quickly to the core of the topic. Biases of the interviewer should not be expressed in the focus group. A special relationship with a specific individual, an affirmative nod at something of which the interviewer approves, or a lack of encouragement for unexpected or unwelcome answers, may bias the interviews. Although conflicts of opinion can produce valuable data, the interviewer must defuse personal hostility between members. Gestures and facial expressions have to be controlled to show members of the group that the interviewer is non-judgmental and values the views of all participants.

The analysis of qualitative focus group interviews

Although there are a variety of different types of analysis for these interviews (Krueger, 1994), the principles of qualitative data analysis are similar to those of other non-structured or semi-structured interviews. Most often the interviews are recorded, and the researcher listens several times to each tape before making transcripts. Although this method has been used in market research, it is difficult to identify individuals' voices on a tape. The problem of identification might be overcome with a video tape.

All tapes, fieldnotes and memos are dated and labelled. A wide margin is left on the transcript for coding and categorising. The transcription should include laughter, notes about pauses and emphasis, and the researcher should make field notes on anything unusual, interesting or contradictory and write memos about theoretical ideas while listening, transcribing and reading. It is important to be clear about who says what, because this can identify those individuals who try to dominate the discussion. The interviewer could note this down while listening to the tape. At the listening stage, major themes and patterns can already be found.

Interviewers code paragraphs and sentences by extracting the essence of ideas within them and using labels which they put into the margin of the transcript. Through a reduction of these codes into larger categories, themes and ideas will be found. Krueger (1994) claims that not all data deserve to be of equal importance. The researcher searches for priorities and important themes from the vast amount of data. This method of analysis is similar to those of other approaches, in fact, focus groups can be analysed by grounded theory analysis or a simpler form of latent content analysis. Latent content analysis (Field & Morse, 1985; Wilson, 1989) identifies themes and patterns without using the progressive focusing and theoretical sampling approaches of grounded theory.

The analyst repeats this process with each focus group interview and compares the transcripts. The major themes arising from each interview are then connected with each other; topics in one interview will overlap with those of other focus groups. Once these themes have been formulated, the patterns described and their meaning interpreted, the literature connected with these ideas is discussed. The appropriate literature becomes part of the data as in other qualitative research. Researchers substantiate their work with relevant quotes from the participants, showing the data from which the patterns and constructs arise.

To write up the study, the interviewer develops a storyline, that is, he or she produces an account which must be readable and clear. The main concerns of the participants have to emerge from the report as the most important parts of the story.

Strengths and limitations of focus groups

In general the advantages and limitations in this approach are those of all qualitative interviews, but there are a number of strengths and weaknesses specific to focus groups (Stewart & Shamdasani, 1990; Morgan 1988; Krueger 1994). The main strength is the production of data through social interaction. The dynamic inter-action stimulates the thoughts of participants and reminds them of their own feelings about the research topic. Informants build on the answers of others in the group.

Secondly, on responding to each others' comments, informants might generate new and spontaneous ideas which researchers had not thought of before or during the interview. Through interaction they remember forgotten feelings and thoughts. Thirdly, all the participants, including the interviewer, have the opportunity to ask questions, and these will produce more ideas than individual interviews. Informants can build on the answers of others. Kitzinger (1994) maintains that the group interaction gives courage to the informants to mention even sensitive topics.

The interviewer has the opportunity for prompts and questions for clarification just like the other members of the group. These probes will produce more ideas than individual interviews, and the answers show the participants' feelings about a topic and the priorities in the situation under discussion. The researcher can clarify conflicts between participants and ask about the reasons for these differing views. Focus groups produce more data in the same space of time; this could make them cheaper and quicker than individual interviews.

There are also some disadvantages. The researcher generally has more difficulty managing the debate and less control than in one-to-one interviews. As group members interact throughout the interview, one or two individuals may dominate the discussion and influence the outcome or perhaps even introduce bias as the other members may be merely compliant. The group effect may, as Carey & Smith (1994) suggest, lead to conformity or to convergent answers. They use the term 'censoring', by which they mean the critical stance of group members towards each other. The participants affect each other, while in individual interviews the *real* feelings of the individual informant may be more readily revealed.

A person who is unable to verbalise feelings and thoughts will not make a good informant. Indeed, Merton & King (1990) stress the importance of educational homogeneity of the group. If group members have similar educational back-grounds, the chance for contribution from all members is greater. The status of a few well-educated individuals would inhibit the rest of the members in the group and might even silence them, and therefore similarity of social background is useful. This means that sampling procedures which determine the composition of the group are of paramount importance.

The group climate can inhibit or fail to stimulate an individual or it can, of course, be stimulating and lively and generate more data. Where a researcher feels certain that confrontation and conflict is likely to occur between potential group members, she or he has to be sensitive to group feelings and reconcile their ideas. Conflict can be destructive but can also generate rich data. In any conflict situation, ethical issues must be carefully considered.

Krueger (1994) suggests that researchers experience greater difficulty getting groups together at a certain time and location, while finding it easy to make appointments with individuals. Transcription can be much more difficult because peoples' voices vary, and the distance they sit from the microphone influences the clarity of individuals' contributions. As there are certain dangers of group effect and group member control, it is useful to analyse the interviews both at group level and at the level of the individual participants. The researcher must remember that the data are located within the context of the group setting (Carey & Smith, 1994). Field notes should be made immediately after the session.

Summary

A focus group consists of a small number of people with common experiences or areas of interest. Several focus groups are involved in each study. Whilst the interviews are carefully planned, the interviewer must at the same time be flexible and non-judgmental.

The dynamic of the group situation is intended to stimulate ideas and elicit feelings about the focus of the study. It is important that an open climate exists so that group members feel comfortable about sharing their thoughts and feelings. The data can be analysed by any of the major methods of qualitative analysis.

References

Carey M.A. (1994) The group effect in focus groups: planning, implementing and interpreting focus group research. In *Critical Issues in Qualitative Research Methods* (ed. J.M. Morse), pp. 225–241, Sage, Thousand Oaks, California.

Carey M.A. & Smith M.W. (1994) Capturing the group effect in focus groups. *Qualitative Health Research*, **4**(1), 123–127.

Dignan M. *et al.* (1990) The role of focus groups in health education for cervical cancer among minority women. *Journal of Community Health*, **15**(6), 369–375.

Field P.A. & Morse J.M. (1985) *Nursing Research: The Application of Qualitative Approaches.* Croom Helm, London.

Greenbaum T.L. (1988) *The Practical Handbook and Guide to Focus Group Research.* Lexington Books, D.C. Heath, Lexington.

Hart G. & Rotem A. (1990) Using focus groups to identify clinical learning opportunities for registered nurses. *The Australian Journal of Advanced Nursing*, **8**(1), 16–21.

Kingry J.M., Tiedje L.B. & Friedman L.L. (1990) Focus groups: a research technique for nursing. *Nursing Research*, **39**(2), 124.

Kitzinger J. (1994) The methodology of focus groups: the importance of interaction between research participants *Sociology of Health & Illness*, **16**(1), 102–121.

Krueger R.A. (1994) *Focus Groups: A Practical Guide for Applied Research* 2nd edn. Sage, Thousand Oaks, California.

Merton R.K. & Kendall P.L. (1946) The focused interview. *American Journal of Sociology*, **51**, 541–557.

Merton R.K. & King R. (1990) *The Focused Interview: A Manual of Problems and Procedures* 2nd edn. Free Press, New York.

Morgan D.L. (1988) *Focus Groups as Qualitative Research.* Sage, Newbury Park, California.

Morgan D.L. & Krueger R. A. (1993) When to use focus groups and why. In *Successful Focus Groups: Advancing the State of the Art* (ed. D.L. Morgan), pp.3–19, Sage, Newbury Park, California.

Morgan D.L. & Spanish M.T. (1985) Social interaction and the cognitive organisation of health-relevant knowledge. *Sociology of Health and Illness*, **7**(3), 401–422.

Nyamati A. & Shuler P. (1990) Focus group interview: a research technique for informed nursing practice. *Journal of Advanced Nursing*, **15**, 1281–1288.

Patton M. (1990) *Qualitative Evaluation and Research Methods* 2nd edn. Sage, Newbury Park, California.

Ratcliffe B. (1994) Post-operative nurse–patient interaction during 'patient controlled analgesia'. Unpublished MSc dissertation, University of Surrey, Guildford.

Stewart D.W.& Shamdasani P.N. (1990) *Focus Groups, Theory and Practice.* Sage, Newbury Park, California.

Wilson H.S. (1989) The craft of qualitative analysis. In *Research in Nursing* (ed. H.S. Wilson), pp. 394–428, Addison-Wesley, Menlo Park, California.

Chapter 11

Additional Approaches

This chapter outlines the following approaches:

- Conversation analysis
- Qualitative action research
- Qualitative case study research

Some other approaches are briefly mentioned

Conversation analysis

Within the great variety of qualitative methods, some emphasise language and language use. Any professional–client interaction relies on the use of language as a major communication device. Conversation(al) analysis (CA) is a form of discourse analysis which examines the use of language and asks the question of how everyday conversation works (Nunan, 1993). This type of enquiry focuses on ordinary conversations and on the way in which talk is organised and ordered in speech exchanges. While researchers primarily examine speech patterns, they also analyse non-verbal behaviour in interaction, such as mime, gesture and other body language. As Nofsinger (1991:2) explains: 'If we are to understand interpersonal communication, we need to learn how this is accomplished so successfully'.

The origins of conversation analysis (CA)

CA was initially developed in the 1960s and 1970s in the United States by Harold Garfinkel, Harvey Sacks, Emmanuel Schegloff and others. While other types of discourse analysis have their roots in the field of linguistics, CA originates in ethnomethodology, a specialist direction of sociology and phenomenology. Ethnomethodology focuses in particular on the world of social practices, interactions and rules (see Turner, 1974). Garfinkel attempted to uncover the ways in which members of society construct social reality.

Ethnomethodologists focus on the practical accomplishments of members of society, seeking to demonstrate that these make sense of their actions on the basis of *tacit knowledge*, their shared understanding of the rules of interaction. Goodwin & Heritage (1990:283) summarise this: 'through processes of social interaction, shared meaning, mutual understanding and the coordination of human conduct are achieved'.

The use of CA

CA focuses on what individuals say in their everyday conversation, but also on what they do (Nofsinger, 1991). Through conversation, movement and gesture, we learn of people's intentions and ideas. The sequencing and turn-taking in conversations demonstrate the meaning individuals give to situations and show how they inhabit a shared world. Body movements too, are the focus of analysis. Conversation analysts do not use interviewing to collect data but analyse ordinary talk, 'naturally occurring' conversations. Most sections of talk which they analyse are relatively small, and the analysis is detailed. According to Heritage (1988:130) CA makes the assumptions that talk is 'structurally organised', and each turn of talk is influenced by the context of what has gone on before and establishes another context, towards which the next turn will be oriented.

CA is more often used in sociological or education studies rather than in nursing. We think though that it could be a valuable research approach in nursing and lead to changes in the interaction between nurses and patients or other health professionals. Researchers generally audio- or video-tape these interactions and trancribe the conversations in a particular way (see transcription techniques in Nofsinger, 1991, or, in more detail in Button & Lee, 1987) largely developed by Gail Jefferson.

Example of CA

A good example of the use of CA is given by Couchman (personal communication, 1995) who used a piece of action research to train staff working with people who have learning difficulties. Video-taping staff and clients in day centres she found that staff had underestimated the responsiveness of clients and did not always notice their readiness for interaction. When shown the tapes staff became more aware of clients' needs and responded quickly.

There are examples in nursing research of doctor–patient or nurse–patient interaction which show how talk is generated and organised by the participants and follows an orderly process in which a turn-taking system exists (Sharrock & Anderson, 1987; Bergstrom et al., 1992). Tapes show what actually takes place in a setting.

Example

Mallett (1990) explored the interaction between nurses and post-anaesthetic patients. She video-taped dental patients post-operatively. Verbal and non-verbal communication was observed. Mallett found that nurses varied in the ways in which they engaged with patients, depending on their needs and level of consciousness. She highlighted some of the difficulties in the situation and indicated how the analysis of nurse–patient interactions could illustrate potential problems and could be used as a teaching aid for novices.

The analysis of CA includes the discovery of regularities in speech or body movement, the search for deviant cases and the integration with other findings without over-generalisation (Heritage, 1988). One of the disadvantages is the way in which conversation analysts emphasise the formal characteristics of interaction at the expense of content, but they do focus on the dynamic aspects in which interaction takes place (Leudar & Antaki, 1988).

CA is difficult, highly complex and very detailed. Researchers may not find it easy, and we would not recommend it to novice researchers.

Action research

One of the most useful and frequent types of research in nursing is action research. Researchers who use this method believe in creating change in the setting they investigate (Hart & Bond, 1995). In nursing this means the identification of a specific problem in clinical or educational practice and trying to change this with the aim of improving the situation. Webb (1991:155) states that 'action research is a way of doing research and working on problems at the same time'. It generally involves small-scale intervention in a setting, process or treatment, and an evaluation or review of the impact of this process. Nursing has always been linked to intervention and change; any health worker's aim is to change the condition or illness of individual patients or the health status of a particular group. Because of its small scale the research is generally, though not always, qualitative.

The historical background

Action research has its origin in the educational problem-solving approach of the 1940s in the USA; its first well-known exponent was Kurt Lewin (1890–1947), the social psychologist. Lewin (1946) suggested a circular process for action research which includes planning, executing and fact-finding for evaluation. It has also been used in industry and health care. Members of the Tavistock Institute developed their own action research with its basis in psychology and psychoanalysis. Modern nurse researchers have translated Lewin's ideas into a framework with several stages: planning, acting, observing and reflecting (Meyer, 1993). The common aims of action researchers were to change practice, to evaluate this change, act upon it, and to develop and modify theory.

The nature of action research and its use in nursing

Holter & Schwartz-Barkott (1993) give four characteristics of action research:

(1) Collaboration between researcher and practitioner
(2) Solution of practical problems
(3) Change in practice
(4) Development of theory

These four elements are necessary for successful action research. Without colla-boration from the people in the setting, changes in practice cannot be made. These changes are seen as necessary to solve problems. Without development of theory, the research stays arid.

Action research in nursing generally involves a researcher and participants in a clinical or educational situation and is called participatory action research (PAR). Planning action involves an objective which researchers seek to achieve in colla-boration with people in the clinical setting. PAR thus involves those who work in the setting; the traditional roles of researcher and practitioner are broken down. Practitioners become co-researchers. An example of this is given in the paper by Titchen & Binnie (1993).

Example

Titchen & Binnie (1993) started a piece of action research at the John Rad-cliffe Hospital in Oxford. The aim of the research study was to help staff nurses on two wards to change from traditional to patient-centred nursing. The main participants were a researcher with a physiotherapy background and a senior sister. The latter involved the ward sisters with whom she shared identification of problems and decision-making processes. The changes were carried out by the people in the setting, and reflected on and evaluated by them in collaboration with the researcher.

In this study the practitioner as insider became co-researcher with the outsider. Roles between co-researchers are continually negotiated. This prevents burdening the practitioner with too much clinical work or the initial researcher with too much writing and analysing.

Case studies

The term *case study* is used for a variety of research approaches, both qualitative and quantitative. Most qualitative research could be seen as case study research, but we would like to argue that it differs from other qualitative approaches because of its specific focus. A case study is an entity which is studied as a single unit and it has clear boundaries. Merriam (1988:9) defines it as 'an examination of a specific phenomenon, such as a program, an event, a person, a process, an institution, or a social group'. The boundaries of the case should be clarified in terms of the questions asked, the data sources used and the setting and person(s) involved. Although different authors have their own definitions and ideas about the nature of the case study, they also agree on many issues (Platt, 1988).

Case studies can be quantitative, qualitative or both, but we shall summarise here the main features of the qualitative case study which tends to be more common in nursing research. It is often combined with action research (Webb, 1989).

Background

The case study is used in a number of disciplines such as anthropology, sociology or geography, though not all studies of limited cases are case studies. It has been most popular in business studies, but is also used in social work and nursing.

The best known writer on this type of research, Robert Yin, has discussed case studies in a number of books and articles (for example, Yin, 1993, 1994). Although his writing, on the whole, focuses on the quantitative framework, he sees the qualitative approach as valid.

Example of case study

One of the most famous early case studies is that of Whyte (1943) in which he studied a neighbourhood gang in Chicago. Other researchers who used ideas from this study found that it was a 'typical case', meaning that theories emerging from this work could be applied to their research.

Features and purpose of case study research

Generally, nurse researchers who develop case studies are familiar with the case they study and its context before the start of the research. Nurses study a case because they may be interested in it for professional reasons or because they need the knowledge about the particular case.

As in other types of qualitative research, the case study is a way of exploring the phenomenon or phenomena in their context. The researchers, therefore, use a number of sources in their data collection, for instance observation, documentary sources and interviews, so that the case can be illuminated from all sides. Observation and documentary research are the most common strategies used in case study research. It does not have specific methods for data collection or analysis; for instance, the researcher can apply ethnographic or phenomenological approaches. The analysis of qualitative case studies involves the same techniques as that of other qualitative methods: the researcher categorises, develops typologies and generates theoretical ideas.

Studies focus on individuals such as a patient or a group which might consist of individuals with common experiences or characteristics, a ward or a hospital. Life histories of individuals would also be interesting examples of cases.

Examples

In the community, a researcher might shadow district nurses throughout the day and explore their interaction with a specific group such as patients with leg ulcers.

In a children's ward, the nurse researcher could explore all specialist nurses' work and their interaction with children at the time of the doctors' round.

In nursing studies with a psychological emphasis, cases often focus on individuals and an aspect of their behaviour, while the nurse sociologist is more interested in groups. Kent (1992) sees an institution as a case. She examined multiple cases – organisations which provided midwifery education. Her 'case' focused on both the physical and social elements in the setting.

As in other qualitative research, case studies explore the phenomenon or phenomena under study in their context, indeed Platt (1988) states that case studies are holistic and contextual. The lines of division between the phenomena and the context, however, are not always clear (Yin, 1994).

Case studies can be exploratory devices, for instance they may be a pilot for a larger study or for more quantitative research, they could also illustrate the specific elements of a research project. One of our students demonstrated all the ideas which she obtained from informants by writing up the case of one single participant. Usually the case study stands on its own and involves intensive observation. The description of specific cases can make a study more lively and interesting.

Case study research is used mainly to investigate cases which are tied to a specific situation and locality, and hence this type of enquiry is even less readily generalisable than other qualitative research. Therefore researchers are often advised to study typical and multiple cases (Stake, 1995). Atypical cases may, however, sometimes be interesting because their very difference might illustrate the typical case. It is important though that the researcher does not make unwarranted assertions on the basis of a single case.

Meier & Pugh (1986) argue that clinical knowledge improves through focusing on individual cases which nurses collect, be they about responses of the individual to illness or to treatment and interventions. Meier & Pugh stress the importance of a detailed decision trail so that other cases can be studied in the light of the findings of a single case.

Other approaches

The approaches mentioned above are not exclusive, other styles of qualitative research do exist, but they are less common in nursing. *Historical research* is used frequently and *repertory grid methods* are adopted occasionally, particularly in nurse education. So-called *new paradigm research* has also been tried by nurse researchers. *Discourse analysis* is used in studies which have psychological and sociological elements.

Historical research can be qualitative, it often starts without firm assumptions and preconceived ideas. Researchers might, for instance, study a particular era in history or attempt to find out how a particular condition was treated.

Example

One of our colleagues, a midwifery tutor, studied the social construction of episiotomy over the last 150 years. She immersed herself in the literature and analysed the changes in attitudes and techniques which had occurred in this time, and the ways in which professional power had influenced this treatment.

(Way, 1995)

Historical research generally means analysing contemporary texts and documentary sources and books by experts who discuss the period of history or the condition under study. Newspapers and archives too, supply useful information. Primary sources provide the best data and first hand accounts (Fitzpatrick, 1993); they have not undergone the same process of interpretation, although the originator, too, has influenced what is written. Often the researcher attempts to develop a comparison between past and present. It is useful in nursing to apply the insights gained through studying the past.

The psychology of personal constructs, or the repertory grid technique is sometimes seen as qualitative. George Kelly, a psychologist, was the originator and developer of this approach (Kelly, 1955, 1986; Beail 1985). The emphasis is on the idea of 'man (sic) the scientist', that is, individuals themselves give meaning to their action and make sense of the world, and on the basis of this they predict that something will or will not happen. Kelly argues that people are unique in building a framework of constructs on the dimensions of similarity and differences. This approach has been used especially in nurse education, psychiatric nursing and clinical psychology (Banister *et al.*, 1994; Rawlinson, 1995).

Participatory action research is an example of co-operative research. Another form of co-operative research was developed by Reason and Rowan (Reason & Rowan, 1981; Reason, 1988) which they called new paradigm research. So-called new paradigm research can include many types of qualitative enquiry, but it differs in some respects. In this approach, researchers and informants are active participants in the process and all decide on the methods and meanings. It is closely connected with humanistic psychology and the work of John Heron and his colleagues, as well as the tradition of critical theory. It also has similarities with feminist research methodologies. This type of research abolishes the division between researcher and researched which is not often stipulated in conventional qualitative research texts.

Discourse analysis, used by sociologists and psychologists, is the study of language in use (Nunan, 1993:7). Researchers familiar with this type of analysis examine a text or a narrative. The purpose of this is to identify patterns and regularities and to uncover the meanings contained in the discourse. Discourse analysis, like conversation analysis, gives more specific attention to minute detail than other qualitative approaches.

It would go too far to discuss any of these approaches in detail, nor can we mention all types of possible qualitative enquiry. The major qualitative approaches at present which are taken by nursing students and researchers are discussed in detail in the main part of this book.

Summary

This chapter gives an overview of a number of lesser known or less often used qualitative research methods, such as conversation and discourse analysis. Action research and case study research can be both qualitative and quantitative but are often adopted by qualitative nurse researchers. Historical approaches, personal construct methods and so-called new paradigm research are also mentioned, but this chapter's aim is merely to show that approaches exist which have not been discussed in detail.

References

For conversation analysis

Antaki C. (1988) *Analysing Everyday Explanation: A Casebook of Methods*. Sage, London.

Bergstrom L., Roberts J., Skillman L. & Seidel J. (1992) You'll feel me touching you, sweetie: vaginal examination during the second stage of labour. *Birth*, **19**, 11–18.

Button G. & Lee J.R.E. (1987) *Talk and Social Organization*. Multilingual Matters, Clevedon.

Goodwin C. & Heritage J. (1990) Conversation analysis. *Annual Review of Anthropology*, **19**, 283–307.

Heritage J. (1988) Explanations as accounts: a conversation analytic perspective. In *Analysing Everyday Explanation: A Casebook of Methods* (ed. C. Antaki), pp. 127–144, Sage, London.

Leudar I. & Antaki C. (1988) Completion and dynamics in explanation seeking. In *Analysing Everyday Explanation: A Casebook of Methods* (ed. C. Antaki), pp. 145–155, Sage, London.

Mallett J. (1990) Communication between nurses and post-anaesthetic patients. *Intensive Care Nursing*, **6**, 45–53.

Nofsinger R.E. (1991) *Everyday Conversation*. Sage, Newbury Park, California.

Nunan D. (1993) *Discourse Analysis*. Penguin, Harmondsworth.

Sharrock W. & Anderson R. (1987) Work flow in a paediatric clinic. In *Talk and Social Organisation* (eds G. Button & J.R.E. Lee), Multilingual Matters, Clevedon.

Turner R. (1974) *Ethnomethodology*. Penguin Books, Harmondsworth.

For action research

Hart E. & Bond M. (1995) *Action Research for Health and Social Care*. Open University Press, Milton Keynes.

Holter I.M. & Schwartz-Barcott D. (1993) Action research: What is it? How has it been used, and how can it be used in nursing? *Journal of Advanced Nursing*, **18**, 298–304.

Lewin K. (1946) Action research and minority problems. *Journal of Social Issues*, **2**, 34–46.

Meyer J.E. (1993) New paradigm research in practice: the trials and tribulations of action research. *Journal of Advanced Nursing*, **18**, 1066–1072.

Titchen A. & Binnie A. (1993) Collaborative action research in nursing. *Journal of Advanced Nursing*, **18**, 858–865.

Webb C. (1989) Action research: philosophy, methods and personal experiences. *Journal of Advanced Nursing*, **14**, 403–410.

Webb C. (1991) Action research. In *The Research Process in Nursing* 2nd edn (ed. D.F.S. Cormack), pp. 155–165, Blackwell Science, Oxford.

For case studies

Kent J. (1992) An evaluation of pre-registration midwifery education in England. *Midwifery*, **8**, 69–75.

Meier P. & Pugh E.J. (1986) The case study: a viable approach to clinical research. *Research in Nursing and Health*, **9**, 195–202.

Merriam S.J. (1988) *Case Study Research in Education*. Jossey Bass, San Francisco.

Platt J. (1988) What can case studies do? *Studies in Qualitative Methodology*, **1**, 2–23.

Stake R.E. (1995) *The Art of Case Study Research*. Sage, Thousand Oaks, California.

Webb C. (1989) Action research: philosophy, methods and personal experiences. *Journal of Advanced Nursing* **14**, 403–410.

Whyte W.F. (1943) *Street Corner Society: The Social Structure of an Italian Slum*. University of Chicago Press, Chicago.

Yin R.K. (1993) *Applications of Case Study Research*. Sage, Newbury Park, California.

Yin R.K. (1994) *Case Study Research* 2nd edn. Sage, Thousand Oaks, California.

Other approaches

Banister P., Bruman E., Parker I., Taylor M. & Tindall C. (1994) *Qualitative Methods in Psychology: A Research Guide*. Open University, Milton Keynes.

Beail N. (1985) *Repertory Grid Technique and Personal Constructs: Applications in Clinical and Educational Settings*. Croom Helm, London.

Fitzpatrick M.L. (1993) Historical research: the method. In *Nursing Research: A Qualitative Perspective* (eds P. Munhall & C. Oiler Boyd), pp. 359–371, National League for Nursing Press, New York.

Kelly G. (1955) *A Theory of Personality: The Psychology of Personal Constructs* Volumes 1 and 2. Norton, New York.

Kelly G. (1986) *A Brief Introduction into Personal Construct Theory*. Centre for Personal Construct Theory, London.

Nunan D. (1993) *Discourse Analysis*. Penguin English, London.

Rawlinson J.W. (1995) Some reflections on the use of repertory grid technique in studies of nurses and social workers. *Journal of Advanced Nursing*, **21**, 334–339.

Reason P. (1988) *Human Inquiry in Action*. Sage, London.

Reason P. & Rowan J. (1981) *Human Inquiry: A Sourcebook of New Paradigm Research*. Wiley, Chichester.

Way S. (1995) Episiotomy: a review of the historical and contemporary literature. Unpublished MSc dissertation, University of Surrey, Guildford.

In this chapter we discuss:

- Early issues concerning rigour in qualitative research
- Criteria for establishing trustworthiness in qualitative research

All research is rightly open to criticism, and there must be criteria by which qualitative research can be evaluated. For quantitative research, objectivity is one of the most important criteria by which the research is judged. It contains two parts: validity and reliability (Minichiello *et al.* 1990). As research findings have implications for practice, these findings cannot be implemented without first thorough examination of the objectivity of the research itself. Validity is the extent to which any research tool measures what it is supposed to do. Reliability is the extent to which an instrument, when used more than once, will produce the same results or answer in research.

Clarke (1995) argues that some qualitative methodologists try to achieve academic standing by applying the terms and concepts used in quantitative approaches. Indeed, Brink (1991) claims that these terms linger in qualitative research because reviewers of articles (and, we may add, members of grant holding bodies) are still, in the main, knowledgeable about quantitative methods but less informed about qualitative research.

We would argue that issues concerning validity and reliability are different in qualitative research (Wheeler, 1992). Indeed, we suggest that researchers do not use these terms in qualitative enquiry as different criteria and concepts have been introduced. Guba & Lincoln (1985), for instance, use the term *trustworthiness* instead of validity. Trustworthiness exists when the findings of a qualitative study represent reality.

Early issues concerning rigour in qualitative research

Qualitative research has elements of subjectivity. In 1986 Munhall & Oiler argued that, whilst tension exists between the so-called *subjective human reality* (the inner private world) and *objective human reality* (the outer observable world), these concepts are not mutually exclusive. In fact they prefer to bring these together and state:

'In the view of the qualitative researcher, subjective experience is not merely a private inner world, but rather inextricably bound with objective reality and the basis from which scientific knowledge is derived.'

This is an important statement for the evaluation of qualitative research because it acknowledges that objective reality and subjective experiences potentially exist together in the research data. Qualitative research projects therefore require different approaches to validity and reliability and different concepts. These need to be both clear and demonstrable throughout the study. The researcher must show that the study is rigorous by establishing trustworthiness (Sandelowski, 1986; Koch, 1994). The term became an important concept in the examination and critical analysis of qualitative research projects. It is therefore central to the whole research process, where the researcher needs to demonstrate a 'decision trail' (Sandelowski, 1986) that can be followed by other researchers.

The decision trail involves the researcher in presenting, clarifying and justifying both the chosen methodology and the data analysis. Koch (1994) argues that the reader of the report should be able to audit this trail in terms of actions taken by the researcher and any influences (biases) that affect the research. The two elements of rigour, trustworthiness and the decision trail, provide the key issues for both students and supervisors in trying to ensure rigour in qualitative research.

(1) Can the research be audited properly (the trustworthiness established)?
(2) Are the actions of researchers, and influences on them, and events that occurred during the research clearly demonstrated (the decision trail shown)?

One of the early nurse researchers to address these twin concerns was Sandelowski (1986) in a seminal paper. She argued that prior to this there were few discussions in the literature about how to ensure that qualitative research was rigorous, yet faithful and relevant to nursing perspectives. Sandelowski claimed that the debate was complicated by the argument that qualitative research should be evaluated by the same criteria of conventional, scientific rigour as other types (Chalmers, 1982, however, points out that the so-called scientific approach is not itself without problems). Sandelowski developed the classic paper for qualitative nursing research, which formed the basis for establishing and ensuring rigour.

Criteria for establishing trustworthiness

Guba & Lincoln (1985, 1989) make a case for alternatives to develop effective evaluation of qualitative research. The four alternatives are credibility, transferability, dependability and confirmability. These alternatives provide the foundations for demonstrating both trustworthiness and the decision trail in qualitative research. Most recently they have been supported by the work of a nurse researcher, Koch (1994), who explores the decision trail in detail, using the ideas of Guba & Lincoln (1985, 1989). Robson (1993) presents these factors as alternatives for qualitative researchers.

Credibility

To establish credibility in a study, researchers must ensure that those participating in research are identified and described accurately. According to Koch (1994:977), 'credibility is enhanced when researchers describe and interpret their experience as researchers' thus showing their own involvement.

Example

A registered general nurse and nurse tutor on a part time nursing degree chose to investigate qualified nurses' perceptions of the meaning of care. To enhance credibility the researcher declared and described her own experience of caring thus:

'I experience caring as a nurse to mean a process of "discovering" the other person and interacting within that discovery. To activate personal energy in understanding the person's frame of reference and using empathy to create a relationship of support and concern. As a nurse, I use the skills learnt from professional, practical and theoretical knowledge to facilitate the person through the potentially difficult process of being a patient.'

(Clarke, 1991).

Robson (1993) follows Guba & Lincoln (1985) in suggesting several actions to improve credibility: prolonged involvement, persistent observation, triangulation, peer debriefing and member checks.

Prolonged involvement means spending enough time to learn about the culture and build trust with those participating in the research (the research informants), because they can only be understood when researchers have invested enough time in the setting. In anthropological case studies this is essential as part of the research process, but it is also important for other qualitative research. Persistent observation concerns situations that are studied for enough time to allow for selectivity of what is most relevant and representative for the issues being examined. This type of observation allows for depth in the research.

Triangulation allows the use of different approaches and methods in collecting data. For instance, a researcher could both observe and interview participants, or could use both qualitative and quantitative methods (see also the debate in Chapter 1). Data from one source can be checked against the other.

Example

A student undergraduate nurse investigated attitudes of student nurses towards the subject of passive euthanasia. In this study the researcher decided to combine qualitative and quantitative approaches to investigate attitudes and thereby triangulate (use evidence from different sources). The qualitative

Example *contd.*

part of this research consisted of four in-depth interviews with student nurses to gain an initial insight into their perceptions, thoughts and feelings, towards passive euthanasia. The interview data provided a precursor for developing the research.

The themes and categories that emerged in the analysis were linked with the subsequent literature. Certain hypotheses were constructed from these data which were tested by constructing vignettes. The quantitative part of the research concerned presenting those vignettes to a further sample of student nurses using a questionnaire which incorporated a Likert Scale for rating responses (Ingram, 1994).

Peer debriefing concerns presenting data analysis and conclusions for peer evaluation. Supervisors who have the skills for the particular research approach are necessary for this role. Undergraduate student nurses and higher degree students need to meet regularly during the research process with their designated supervisor, to ensure rigour in their projects (see Chapter 16).

Member checks, advocated by Lincoln & Guba (1985), involve those who participated in the research (the sample) in checking the research findings to make sure that they are true to their experience. Robson (1993) suggests that this would be a direct way of improving the credibility of the study. Yet he warns that if an individual or group who participated in the study has an interest in misrepresenting the findings (because of possible closure of a unit in a hospital or other consideration) member bias may occur, and researchers must be aware of this. Nurse researchers might also discuss the findings of the study with their colleagues who would bring a fresh perspective on the research.

An interesting example of involving research informants occurs in the Colaizzi (1978) seven-stage approach for phenomenological data analysis. The seventh stage of this analysis requires the researcher to take the descriptive results to those informants who took part in the study (the sample) for validation. The research informants compare the descriptive results with their experience as lived.

Example

In the study concerning qualified nurses' perceptions of the meaning of care (mentioned above) the inductive, descriptive research methodology of phenomenology was used in the investigation. The data were analysed using the Colaizzi (1978) seven-stage procedure. The exhaustive description was taken back to the informants for validation rather than the essential structure (final result of data analysis) because the former was deemed to reflect the informants' experiences in a more recognisable form for them to comment on and identify with.

Example *contd.*

The researcher contacted all six informants of this study to obtain agreement for returning to discuss the exhaustive description. With consent, the informants were interviewed using an interview guide adapted from Colaizzi (1978) which concerned four main questions. Informants were asked:

- Do you recognise any of your experiences in this exhaustive description of 'caring'?
- Does it have meaning for you?
- Does it have meaning for caring? For nursing?
- What aspects of your experience or your existence have I omitted?

Research informants were able to respond to these questions when reading the full account of the 'lived experience' of the phenomenon of care contained in the exhaustive description. The researcher then developed the essential structure (final stage of analysis) following informants' suggestions (Clarke & Wheeler, 1992).

Transferability

Transferability is the next criterion for ensuring rigour in research. This is about how the findings can be generalised or transferred from a representative sample of a population to the whole group. In quantitative research, Robson (1993) highlights that this is undertaken within certain rules concerning statistical inference. For qualitative research, however, this is inappropriate because the process of sampling is quite different. Field & Morse (1985) examine this difference in terms of purpose. For quantitative research, the importance is to find out the distribution of phenomena in a population, whereas in qualitative research the purpose is to try and understand the phenomenon, which may not be distributed evenly in a population.

Field & Morse (1985) suggest that the qualitative researcher should state the characteristics and settings of those participating in the research. Morse (1991) discussed the main sampling types in qualitative research: purposeful, nominated, volunteer and total population samples. For purposeful samples, the researcher selects participants that fulfil the study needs. For example, participants may be selected because they have had previous experience of the phenomenon or general knowledge of it.

> ## Example
>
> An undergraduate student nurse wanted to explore the lived experience of chronic illness. In considering the potential sample, she reflected on her experiences with individuals who had multiple sclerosis. The Multiple Sclerosis Society estimate that there are 80 000 people with this condition in the United Kingdom (MS Society, 1992). This gave even more justification for undertaking such a study within the chronic illness context. In selecting participants for the study, obviously the important criterion was the experience of having multiple sclerosis. The sample the student sought became, therefore, a purposeful one (Lodi, 1994).

In nominated or chain referral samples, the researcher gains assistance in selecting other research participants from a single informant.

Volunteer samples are literally those who volunteer to take part in the study following notices and requests. In the notices, adverts and requests used, the researcher asks for particular qualities, e.g. nurses who are first level qualified or clients with a certain condition.

It is our experience of supervising undergraduate studies that in many cases, students request volunteers to participate, provided they have suitable permission, by publishing notices in hospitals and community settings. The total population consists of a sample that involves all those in a setting, for example all the residents of a home or all the members of a family. Morse (1991) points out, however, that for qualitative research this is only possible when the sample is small enough to be manageable.

Whilst these types of sampling are more appropriate for qualitative research, they are not of themselves generalisable or transferable.

The readers have to consider, however, the transferability of the data and findings from a particular study to the general population in a qualitative research project. It is the role of the researcher to aid this by ensuring that the decision trail of the research is clear and comprehensive enough. So, provided a full account of the theoretical framework of the study is given, others using this can then decide if the case or cases described may be transferred to other settings. In effect then, transferability is a part of qualitative research in relationship to specific sampling strategies. Further, judgments are made concerning the transfer of the findings to other settings according to the soundness of the theoretical framework used. The specific knowledge gained in one setting or with one group of people may be transferred to others.

Dependability

Dependability is the third alternative for establishing the trustworthiness of qualitative research and is reliant on credibility. According to Robson (1993) a qualitative research study that establishes credibility will also be dependable. Koch

(1994:977) states: 'One of the ways in which a research study may be shown to be dependable as opposed to consistent, is for its process to be audited', that is, external checks are made. Robson (1993) and Koch (1994) point out that for business an audit involves authenticating the accounts. For research the reader and critic of the research study follows a checking process of the procedures used. If these follow accepted standards and are clear, then the study can be found to be dependable.

The notion of dependability clearly returns to Sandelowski's (1986) concept of the decision trail. In discussing this concept, Koch (1994:978), gives a summary:

'A decision trail provides a means for the researcher to establish audit trail linkages. Leaving a decision trail entails discussing explicitly decisions taken about the theoretical, methodological and analytic choices throughout the study.'

Confirmability

The fourth and last alternative for achieving trustworthiness in a qualitative research study concerns the notion of confirmability. Guba & Lincoln (1989) point out that confirmability means that the data are linked to their sources for the reader to establish that the conclusions and interpretations arise directly from them.

Robson (1993:406) suggests that criteria for auditing the study should involve examining the following information:

- The raw data themselves, e.g. tape recordings, field notes and diaries.
- The analysed data, e.g. findings of the study.
- The formation of the findings, e.g. significant statements, themes, codes and categories.
- The process of this study, e.g. design strategies and procedures used.
- The early intentions of the study, for instance the proposal and expectations.
- The development of the measure(s) used, e.g. open ended questions, early interviews and observation strategies.

Koch (1994) points out that when auditing qualitative research, confirmability occurs with credibility, transferability and dependability as initially suggested by Guba & Lincoln (1989).

These four components for achieving trustworthiness in a qualitative research study provide a logical background for both designing and undertaking a project. Further we support the very important concept of the *decision trail* which allows researchers to process the research and the reader to understand the decisions made. The decision trail provides a way of establishing rigour in qualitative research and auditing (evaluating) the entire study.

It must be remembered that particular qualitative approaches for establishing the trustworthiness of research studies, for instance Strauss & Corbin (1990), give specific guidelines for evaluating grounded theory (see Chapter 7).

Summary

Researchers in qualitative enquiry do not generally use the terms validity and reliability, which are seen as inappropriate. In this type of approach the most common terms are credibility, transferability, dependability and confirmability. Credibility exists when the participants are identified and described accurately. Transferability is judged by the readers of a study after reading the detailed account. They are then able to see whether the case or cases can be transferred to other settings. Dependability is demonstrated if the processes of research are following accepted standards when they are checked. Confirmability is ensured when the reader is able to assess the adequacy of the research process and judge whether the findings come directly from the data.

The researcher must leave a detailed decision or audit trail which enables readers to know how methodological, analytic and theoretical decisions have been made, and helps them to decide on the trustworthiness of the study.

References

Brink P.J. (1991) Dialogue: on issues about reliability and validity. In *Qualitative Nursing Research. A Contemporary Dialogue* (ed. J.M. Morse), p. 163, Sage, Newbury Park, California.

Chalmers A.F. (1982) *What is This Thing Called Science?* 2nd edn. Open University Press, Milton Keynes.

Clarke J. (1991) A view of the phenomenon of caring in nursing practice: a study investigating meaning of caring to practising nurses. Unpublished BSc project, Bournemouth University, Bournemouth.

Clarke L. (1995) Science, vision and telling stories. *Journal of Advanced Nursing*, **21**, 584–593.

Clarke J. B. & Wheeler S. J. (1992) A view of the phenomenon of caring in nursing practice. *Journal of Advanced Nursing*, **17**, 1283–1290.

Colaizzi P. (1978) Psychological research as the phenomenologist views it. In *Existential Phenomenological Alternatives for Psychology* (eds R. Valle & M. King), pp. 48–71, Oxford University Press, New York.

Field P.A. & Morse J.M. (1985) *Nursing Research, The Application of Qualitative Approaches*. Croom Helm, London.

Guba E .G & Lincoln Y.S. (1981) *Effective Evaluation*. Jossey Bass, San Francisco.

Guba E. & Lincoln Y. (1985) *Effective Evaluation: Improving the Usefulness of Evaluation. Results through Responses and Naturalistic Approaches*. Jossey Bass, San Francisco.

Guba E. & Lincoln Y. (1989) *Fourth Generation Evaluation*. Sage, Newbury Park, California.

Ingram R. (1994) Passive euthanasia – the student nurses' perspective. Unpublished BSc study, Bournemouth Unversity, Bournemouth.

Koch T. (1994) Establish rigor in qualitative research: the decision trail. *Journal of Advanced Nursing*, **19**, 976–986.

Lincoln Y.S. & Guba E.G. (1985) *Naturalistic Inquiry*. Sage, Beverly Hills, California.

Lodi Y. (1994) The lived experience of multiple sclerosis: a phenomenological inquiry. Unpublished BSc project, Bournemouth University, Bournemouth.

Minichiello V., Aroni R., Timewell E. & Alexander L. (1990) *In-Depth Interviewing: Researching People*. Longman Cheshire, Melbourne.

Morse J.M. (1991) Strategies for sampling. In *Qualitative Nursing Research: A Contemporary Dialogue* (ed. J.M. Morse), pp. 127–156, Sage, Newbury Park, California.

Munhall P.L. & Oiler C.J. (1986) *Nursing Research, A Qualitative Perspective*. Appleton, Century Crofts, Norwalk, Connecticut.

Robson C. (1993) *Real World Research: A Resource for Social Scientists and Practitioner Researchers*. Blackwell Science, Oxford.

Sandelowski M. (1986) The problem of rigor in qualitative research. *Advances in Nursing Science*, **8**(3), 27–37.

Strauss A. & Corbin J. (1990) *Basics of Qualitative Research: Grounded Theory Procedures and Techniques*. Sage, Newbury Park, California.

Wheeler S.J. (1992) Perceptions of child abuse. *Health Visitor*, **65**, 316–319.

Chapter 13

Writing Up Qualitative Research

In this chapter consideration will be given to the process of writing up the research in the following sequence

- Title, abstract, acknowledgement and contents
- The introduction to the study
- The methodology and research design
- Entry issues and ethical considerations
- The results and discussion
- The story line
- Reflections and conclusion

Researchers submit the results of their studies to others; for instance external examiners, a commissioning or funding agency, or, for peer review, to an academic journal. It is important to be familiar with the format of a research report or dissertation and with general guidelines for its presentation. The research report mirrors the proposal though it is generally more detailed and, of course, includes the findings and discussion. Although conventions for writing up exist, they vary from one institution or agency to another.

Writers must always remember to whom they are addressing the report; there is a clear difference between reports that are written for practitioners in the clinical setting, a report for a major funding body and a research dissertation or thesis. Edwards & Talbot (1994) argue that format and style differ considerably although all reports have commonalities. Employers and practitioners are most interested in the results and implications of the research for practice and less concerned with philosophical and theoretical issues, while editors of academic journals see these as important.

Occasionally nurses feel it is more appropriate to write two separate reports on the research, one for the practice setting, the other for the university in which they are taking their degree. They also write research articles for nursing and academic journals so that the findings can be debated publicly. In a public report for the practice setting or a journal, anonymity and confidentiality of the research participants become major issues as many professionals in the hospital and the community know the patients involved.

The format must fit the design of the research, and there are differences in the writing up between quantitative and qualitative studies. In a qualitative report, the methodology section is of major importance; in fact, Lincoln & Guba (1985) advise researchers to provide an *audit trail*; this means that the methods and logic of the study must be explicit and open to public scrutiny. The biases of the researcher must be stated and laid open to others.

Readers and reviewers should be able to follow all the procedures of the study. Erlandson *et al.* (1993:35) demand that 'an adequate trail should be left ... to determine if the conclusions, interpretations and recommendations can be traced to their sources and if they are supported by the inquiry'. This means that qualitative writing is more reflective than the writing up of other types of research.

The use of the first person

When writing up the introduction and the methodology, researchers use a personalised account (Wolcott, 1990; Webb, 1992). It sounds pompous and arid when they write: the researcher has found ..., the author does ..., the writer considers, etc. Qualitative research, and increasingly quantitative research, does not proceed this way. The researchers can use the first person, *I*, when they mention what they themselves chose to do. For instance, researchers would not say: the author chose a sample, or the researcher used the methods, etc. They may write: I chose a purposive sample of ..., I collected the data through .... It is, of course, important that the *I* is not overused.

In this chapter, we deal primarily with dissertations. Generally, writers of qualitative studies organise their dissertation in the following sequence:

Title
Abstract
Acknowledgement and dedication
Contents
Introduction
    Background and justification of the study
    The aim of the research
    Initial literature review (or overview of the literature)
Ethical considerations
Methodology
    Description and justification of methods
    (including type of theoretical framework such as symbolic interactionism or phenomenology)
    The sample and the setting
    Specific techniques and procedures
    Data analysis
Findings/results and discussion
Conclusion and implications
References
Appendices

It must be remembered that qualitative writing may differ substantially from a quantitative report although commonalities exist. The main distinction lies in the flexibility of the qualitative report. The findings and discussion are the most important elements of the final write-up, and in consequence contain more words.

Title

The title of a study is important, especially if it is presented as a student project, dissertation or thesis, because it is the first and most immediate contact the reader has with the research, and its impact on judging the work can be considerable. We would suggest a concise but informative title which sounds interesting but not facetious. It must be remembered that it is initially a working title and may change when some of the research has been done, so it can encompass emergent ideas. For instance, one of us (Holloway, 1992) decided at the proposal stage, that a piece of research should be entitled: 'The social reality of catering teachers'. After getting halfway through the research when some of the main themes had emerged, it was retitled: 'Dual identities: the social reality of catering teachers'.

Another of us (Wheeler, 1989) examined social workers' and health visitors' perceptions concerning child abuse. This was obviously a lengthy informative title and appropriate for the research project. In the published format, however, the title became 'Perceptions of child abuse' which, whilst not disclosing the background of the research informants, did still capture interest from multi-professionals working in the child protection field (Wheeler, 1992). A title which contains the essence of a qualitative study in nursing was the following: 'We didn't want him to die on his own: nurses' accounts of nursing dying patients' (Field, 1984). Although this title is rather long, it immediately arouses interest.

Another good title is Kramer's (1974) 'Reality shock: why nurses leave nursing'. It can be seen that writers often use explanatory subtitles. Journals and books might generate ideas for titles which capture the reader's attention and imagination.

The title gives a clear picture of the study's content. The methodology need not be included in the title unless it is very unusual. Many students include redundancies in the title such as 'A study of . . .', 'Aspects of . . .', or enquiry, analysis and investigation. A piece of work titled 'A qualitative study of the experience of epilepsy' should become 'The experience of epilepsy'.

Although the title should reflect the aim of the research it would be clumsy to give the whole aim in the title. For instance, 'A study of the needs of relatives of old people with Alzheimer's in long-term hospital care and in the community' would be too long.

The title page in a dissertation or thesis contains the title, the name of the researcher, the date of the dissertation, and the name of the educational institution at which the student was enrolled. There is generally a *pro forma* for the title page at most universities. They specify other details for the finished dissertation such as word allowance or size of margins.

Abstract

The abstract is written last and appears on the page behind the title but before the table of contents and the full report. It summarises the major points of the study and provides the reader with a quick overview of the research question and aim, methods adopted (very brief) and the main results of the study giving brief information on each chapter. From the abstract, readers gain a clear picture of the aim, content, methods and main findings. Depending on the size and type of study, the abstract should contain between 100 and 300 words, usually no more than one sheet of A4 paper in single spacing. Writers should keep to the word limit specified. The abstract is written in the past tense. As not everything can be squeezed in, writers should be selective about the content.

Example of abstract

This qualitative study was designed to gain insight into nurses' perceptions of patients' feelings and needs with specific reference to breast surgery. A grounded theory approach was adopted, based on in-depth unstructured interviews with eight trained nurses working on surgical wards in a district general hospital. It emerged that the informants believed breast surgery patients to be very vulnerable and to be suffering from extreme stress and trauma. Patients were thought to lack knowledge regarding their treatment and condition. The nurses thought it to be their moral and professional duty to act as advocates for the patient and the family. Imposed restrictions on their advocacy role were found to cause a sense of frustration and power-lessness which appeared to be compounded by the nurses' perceived lack of counselling skills and the absence of a readily available counsellor or specialist nurse. Recommendations for improvements in the care of patients under-going breast surgery are based upon these findings.

(Crockford *et al.*, 1993)

Acknowledgement and dedication

Traditionally writers thank those who supported, advised or supervised the research, often researchers gratefully acknowledge the input of the participants. This happens in student projects, PhD theses or books. Sometimes the writing is dedicated to particular individuals such as parents or spouses. Wolcott (1990) claims that researchers sometimes overdo dedications which, he suggests, should only be given in major work, but he does see acknowledgement of others' help as important.

Contents

Most academic studies have a table of contents before the main chapters begin. It cannot, of course, be finished before the whole project is finalised and written. The contents are sectioned into chapter headings and subheadings with page numbers. In an undergraduate student project, the table of contents should be concise and need not be too long and detailed.

Introduction

In the introduction the writer tells the audience about the research question or topic. The introduction consists of the background and context of the research as well as the aim – the overall purpose of the project. Writers explain why they have become interested in the question, how their project relates to the general topic area, and what gap in nursing knowledge might be filled by the new research through linking the question to the possible implications for practice. In the introduction the nurse explains the significance of the study for the clinical setting and how it could improve clinical practice or policy.

Edwards & Talbot (1994:41) tell researchers to give the answers to the following questions. Why this? Why now? Why there? Why me? An introduction to a qualitative study tends to be more personal than introductions to other types of research report. It is important that all the elements of the background section are relevant to the study and set the scene for it. One of our colleagues claims that it is useful for the researcher to ask the 'So what?' question to keep the background section relevant.

Initial literature review (or overview of the literature)

The literature in qualitative studies has a different place from that in quantitative research. Of course it must show some of the relevant research that has been done in the same field. The researchers summarise the main ideas from these studies, some of the problems and contradictions found, and show how they relate to the project in hand. It is important in qualitative reports not to use every piece of known research in the field nor to give a critical review of all the literature, but only the main pertinent studies, including classic and most recent research (Minichiello *et al.* 1990) and the methodological approaches and procedures which were used for them. Gaps in knowledge become apparent at this point. At this stage, the research question is linked to the literature.

By the end of the introductory section, the reader should be in no doubt that a qualitative study, in the form suggested by the researcher, is most appropriate to meet the research aim.

Methodology and research design

The methodology chapter includes several subsections: the research design, including data collection, the sampling, the detailed interviewing or observation procedures, and a description of the data analysis. In qualitative research the methodology takes up more space. It is most important in this type of study because the researcher is the main research tool and has to make explicit the path of the research, so that the reader knows about the details of design, biases, relationships and limitations, and follows the decision trail.

The research design usually includes the main methods. Researchers briefly describe the methodology they adopt and the reasons and justification for it. They also explain the fit between the research question and the methodology.

The sample and setting

The sample is described in detail. As stated before, in qualitative research the purposive sample is not fixed from the beginning. Concepts rather than people are sampled. The writer describes the informants – who they were, how many were chosen and the reasons for the choice. Researchers tell the reader how they obtained their sample and portray the setting in which the study took place. The inclusion of theoretical sampling must be explained.

Example 1: People and setting

In the study five social workers and five health visitors were interviewed. The social workers originated from the same area office, the health visitors came from the same health authority. They also worked in a locale that was coterminous. This was deemed important in order to reduce the difference between operational styles and policies of both the social service office and the health authority (Wheeler, 1989).

Example 2: Theoretical sampling

For instance: the sample was not predetermined but depended on the concepts which were relevant to the emerging theoretical ideas. It seemed that the 12 women were more compliant than the four men in the sample. This was followed up by interviewing a larger group of men.

Strategies for data collection and analysis

The methodology section gives information about the data collection. The researcher describes the procedures such as interviewing, observation or other strategies which were used and any problems encountered. The outline should not be a general essay on procedures but a step by step description of the work in hand so that the reader can follow it closely. Researchers state reasons for using the particular methodology and research strategies and describe the procedures of collecting data. The reader should know how the data were stored.

> ### Example
>
> The data were collected through unstructured interviews (with an *aide mémoire*) which took place in the informants' own homes and were tape-recorded with their permission. They lasted between 1 and 3 hours. I transcribed the interviews and stored the numbered transcriptions safely away from the list of informants' names. Collection and analysis of data took place at the same time as is usual in grounded theory.

Data analysis

The data analysis needs to be explained, including the ways in which data were coded and categorised and how theoretical constructs were generated from the data. It is useful, and essential in dissertations, to give examples from the study. A detailed account of the chosen type of analysis is required. The audience is entitled to know whether a computer analysis was used.

> ### Example of data analysis section (grounded theory)
>
> Using guidelines based on the initial work by Glaser & Strauss (1967), data were collected and analysed simultaneously. The transcriptions of interviews were coded line by line. The method of analysing data by constant comparison is one of grounded theory's unique features (Strauss & Corbin, 1990) and the content elicited from the data was coded, categorised and constantly compared with the content of earlier data collected, to produce concepts grounded in the data. I followed up theoretical concepts which had relevance to the emerging theory. Comparison with the data and selective sampling of the literature was continued until saturation occurred and no new data emerged.

If this were a dissertation, more detail and examples of each step should be given, so that the audit trail is clearly demonstrated.

Entry issues and ethical considerations

Nurse researchers should describe entry and ethical issues (see Chapters 2 and 3). It must be stated how the participants were approached and how researchers gained permission from gatekeepers, those that are in the position of power to grant access to the setting (managers at various levels, trust and ethics committees). If patients are involved, their consultants or GPs would have to be asked for their permission too. It is important that individual participants cannot be recognised in the report. Last, but most importantly, nurses should make explicit how the ethical principles were followed in the study and how the participants' rights were protected.

Findings and discussion

In qualitative research reports, the findings and discussion are usually integrated (but again, no rigid rule exists about this). Some writers present a brief summary of the results in a diagram, and then discuss each major category (or construct, or theme) in detail. In each chapter the data the researcher collected are discussed first. The relevant literature is integrated into the discussion where it fits best and serves as additional evidence for the particular category or as a problem for discussion.

The use of quotes from participants

Direct quotes from the interviews or excerpts from the field notes are inserted at an appropriate place to show some of the data from which the results emerged. Sandelowski (1994) lists some of the uses of quotes in qualitative studies and suggests that they give insight into people's real experiences and illustrate the arguments. The content of the quotes helps the reader to judge how the results were derived from the data and to establish the credibility of the emerging categories and provide the reader with a means of auditing these.

The writer, of course, must take care that the quotes convey the meanings and feelings of the participant and are directly connected with the discussion which they seek to illustrate. Sandelowski gives importance to both content and style of quote. The direct quotation in the participant's words in a study makes the discussion more lively and dynamic. Long rows of quotes from informants or continuous duplication are not needed. Wolcott (1990:67) suggests 'save the best and drop the rest', but frequent very short quotes make the study look fragmented.

The use of quotations from the literature

Trying to give substance to their own arguments, inexperienced nurse researchers often quote the words of experts. This can interrupt the story line of the research. It is better to avoid a quotation when it can be paraphrased or summarised, with the idea being credited to the originator.

However, when a specific phrase is critical and written by a well-known expert or author of a classic text on the field of study, a quote can be used. Occasionally it does enhance a piece of writing and is appropriate. When using a lengthy quote from books or articles, a page number should be given.

> ## Examples
>
> Wolcott (1990:67) suggests: 'Save the best and drop the rest'.
> Wolcott (1990, p. 67) suggests: 'Save the best and drop the rest'.
> Wolcott (1990) suggests: 'Save the best and drop the rest' (p. 67).

We must warn researchers of two common mistakes. First: researchers often write in a very complex way and use incomprehensible terminology. In their fear of sounding simplistic and unacademic, nurses often complicate and obscure simple and clear issues. It is important to express ideas in clear and unambiguous terms, although they should not, of course, be simplistic. The second flaw is linked to a lack of analysis. It is not enough to simply give a collection of lengthy quotes and to summarise their content. This is not analysis! Researchers have to develop their theoretical ideas and interpretations and they can illustrate them with the relevant quotes from the participants.

Telling the tale

In a qualitative report writers tell a story which should be vivid and interesting as well as credible to the reader. This sometimes means writing and rewriting drafts until a story line can be discerned clearly. Although there may be similarities with journalism or fiction, writers have to keep in mind that these stories have a different purpose, namely to give an accurate and systematic analysis of the data and a discussion of the results. This should not be dry and mechanistic, but must reflect the researcher's involvement. The events, the people and their words and actions should be made explicit, so that readers can experience the situation as real, in a similar way to the researcher.

Reflections on the research

Many academic researchers reflect on their project and take a critical stance to it, usually towards the end of their dissertation or thesis. They demonstrate how the research could be improved, extended or illuminated from another angle. At this point they might point to its limitations and their own biases which they did not make explicit in the main body of the study, and describe some of the problems which they encountered. Not all studies contain this reflective section, and sometimes they are part of the conclusion. Nurses who take a reflective stance could discuss at this point how they have professionally and personally developed and changed through the research. Wolcott (1994) states that this personal approach, rarely adopted in quantitative research, is seen as appropriate in qualitative research.

Qualitative researchers must be aware that a statement about validation of their study by a survey or other quantitative methods might suggest that they are not aware that a qualitative study can stand on its own, has its own validation procedures and cannot be judged from the quantitative researcher's point of view.

Conclusion and implications

Generally studies end with a conclusion. The conclusion is a summary of the results in context. It must be directly related to the results of the specific study, and no new elements (or references) should be introduced here. The conclusion reviews what has been learnt in relation to the aim and the theoretical ideas and propositions that emerged from the study. Dramatic and overly assertive conclusions can be dangerous and pretentious in a small project. Novice researchers seldom generate 'formal theory' or come to significant conclusions; in fact, their research is of 'more modest scope and consequence' (Wolcott, 1994:44). However, this does not mean that the small piece of research has no importance or implications for the clinical area.

In nursing research and other projects in professional settings, the conclusion presents the implications and the recommendations that could be made on the basis of the results. The implications can be integrated into the conclusion, they can be discussed toward its end or they can form a separate section following on from the conclusion. It is important to remember that the implications must be based directly on the results of the study, all too often they seem unrelated to the findings.

References

For academic studies the Harvard system of referencing is most often used, but other formal systems of referencing may be acceptable to the students' supervisors. It is best to find out about this before the start of the study from supervisors, course leaders or handbooks.

The writer should compare the references in the text with the selected bibliography and make sure that every reference is included. We often find that student referencing is incomplete, incorrect or insufficient. Page, the singular, is shortened to p., pages, the plural, to pp. but for journals the pp. or p. is often left out. The title of the book or the name of the journal should be underlined or written in italics. Page numbers are given in the references when an article in a journal is given, or a chapter in an edited book is referenced.

Examples

Wolcott H.F. (1990) *Writing Up Qualitative Research*. Sage, Newbury Park, California.

Morse J.M., Bottorff J.L. & Hutchinson S. (1995) The paradox of comfort. *Nursing Research*, 44(1), 14–19.

May K.A. (1991) Interview techniques in qualitative research. In *Qualitative Nursing Research: A Contemporary Dialogue* (ed. J.M. Morse), pp. 188–209, Sage, Newbury Park, California.

Dane (1990:227) gives the most appropriate advice: 'The three most important aspects of the references section are completeness, accuracy and accuracy'.

Appendices

A list of informants (pseudonyms) – their ages, experience or length of service – is sometimes included by writers (making sure, however, that anonymity is preserved, particularly when they might easily be recognised).

An interview guide and a sample interview transcript in a study that uses interviewing, could be attached as an example for the reader to help in understanding the development of the data collection. Some field notes from observations might be given to demonstrate their use. Appendices depend on the advice given to students and on their own common sense, but there should not be too many sections. Sometimes researchers attach the formal initial letter to participants or an example of the letter of permission. A copy of the letter of approval from the ethical committee should be attached where appropriate. The words in appendices do not count as part of the study.

The appendices are placed at the very end of the study after the bibliography in the order in which they appear in the chronology of the study. For instance, the example of the initial letter to participants would be placed before the exemplar of an interview transcript.

Publishing the research

If the findings are significant, the researcher has the responsibility to disseminate them to a wider group such as colleagues and other health professionals. Sometimes nurses produce a book based on their research (Lawler, 1991; Smith, 1992) or a chapter in an edited book such as that by Morse & Johnson (1991). More often, they attempt to publish an article in a professional or academic journal. The length and style of the article will depend on the type of journal; for instance, articles in the *Journal of Advanced Nursing* are more academic and generally longer than those in the *Nursing Standard* or the *Nursing Times*.

The detailed guidelines for scripts are laid out at the front or the back of the journal. Some journal editors want a very detailed description of the methods adopted (for instance the journal *Midwifery*), others claim that a well-known and widely published methodology, such as grounded theory, can be summarised rather than discussed in great detail (*Sociology of Health and Illness*). Writers must take into account the different styles and guidelines of these journals. As a long research study cannot be fully discussed in article format, researchers choose what to include or exclude. For example, just one chapter, one category or a methodological issue might form the basis of the article.

It is important in an article or a book which reports on qualitative research to write in a lively manner. This can be achieved through a good story line and enhanced through vignettes or excerpts from interviews or field notes, taking into account, of course, that individuals should not be recognised in the descriptions. Good diagrams might clarify some of the aspects of the work. Different journals address different audiences.

Strauss & Corbin (1990) claim that three types of paper are published in journals, intended for different readerships:

(1) For colleagues
(2) For practitioners
(3) For lay readers

For colleagues

There are those colleagues who have a particular interest in the theoretical and methodological framework as well as in the research topic. The *Journal of Advanced Nursing*, *Midwifery* and *Qualitative Health Research* are good examples of journals which publish this type of article. The journal *Qualitative Inquiry* deals exclusively with methodological issues but is not a nursing publication (this and *Qualitative Health Research* are journals published in the USA). *Nurse Education Today* covers educational issues and research in nurse and midwifery education. The *Journal of Nursing Management* is concerned with management issues.

For practitioners

Examples of journals which are intended to assist practitioners are *Nursing Times*, *Nursing Standard* and *Senior Nurse*. There are a great number of others. In these journals one can find articles which describe findings and address the implications of these findings. Often the writers of these articles give an overview of procedures or develop ideas which assist in the understanding of patients.

For the lay reader

Some articles are meant for lay readers. Although most nurse researchers do not write for this readership, occasionally an article in a specialist magazine could actually help members of a group or the general population. For instance, articles on research into hormone replacement therapy in a woman's journal might give information to women, albeit short and non-academic. It is necessary that these articles are written with integrity and factual accuracy.

Critical assessment and evaluation of a qualitative research project

Researchers must be aware that the readers of a research study or report apply certain criteria to judge the quality and credibility of the research and look for particular components in the final write-up. Not all, but some of these are specific to qualitative research. The following are important factors which readers consider when evaluating the study. It would be useful for researchers to examine their own studies in the light of these elements.

The research question
Are the sources of the research problem or question stated clearly?
What is the topic area, and has it been justified?
Is the aim suitable and feasible?
Is the problem appropriate for qualitative research?
Is the title concise and informative?

The abstract
Does it state the aim and describe the methodology?
Does it summarise results and state conclusions?

The literature
Is there an initial overview which gives justification for the study?
Does much of the literature become part of the data?
Are the references comprehensive, relevant and up-to date?

Data collection
What are the types of data collection, and are they appropriate for the study?
How are the data collected, transcribed and stored?

The sample
Does the researcher use purposive (including theoretical) sampling?
Are the criteria for sampling made explicit?
Is the sampling explained adequately?
Is the type and size of sample justified?

Entry and ethical issues
Does the researcher state how the informants were accessed?
Who was approached for permission to access?
Were the rights of participants safeguarded (including their right to withdraw)?
Has the researcher ensured the anonymity of participants?
Are issues of power taken into account?
Has the researcher excluded particularly vulnerable clients?
If these are included in the sample, is this inclusion justified?
Are major ethical issues discussed?

Data analysis
Is the method of analysis identified?
Is the data analysis described (giving examples)?
Is the data analysis systematic and detailed?
Do data collection and analysis interact?
Is the decision trail traced in detail?

The findings
Does the researcher explain the trustworthiness (validity) of the study?
Has the study been taken back to participants for a 'member check'?
Is the explanation appropriate for a qualitative approach?
What does the researcher learn from the research?

Is there a story line or core category?

Has the study met its aim?

Is the conclusion clearly stating what was learnt from the research?

Do the conclusions derive from the data?

Importance to nursing or midwifery

Are the implications for clinical practice discussed?

Do they emerge directly from the study?

Blaxter (1995) produced a draft paper for discussion at the Medical Sociology Conference in which she developed some ideas for the evaluation of qualitative research. She states clearly that the criteria by which to judge qualitative research are different from those of quantitative approaches but also argues for rigour in qualitative research.

Summary

Qualitative research provides more flexibility in writing up than quantitative approaches. Readers should, of course, as said before, be able to follow the decisions made during the process of research. The first sections of the write-up are separated into: introduction (the rationale for the study); an overview of the literature to identify a knowledge gap; and a detailed methodology including a description of the sample, data collection and analysis.

Ethical issues and access must also be described. The findings and discussion are, of course, the major part of the study in which the literature is used as added data. The final section of the study contains the conclusions and implications for the clinical setting. We must stress, in particular, the importance of a lively and interesting story line.

References

Blaxter M. (1995) Paper given at a Workshop on Criteria for the Evaluation of Qualitative Research. Medical Sociology Conference, York, 22–24 September, British Sociological Association.

Crockford E., Holloway I. & Walker J. (1993) Nurses' perceptions of patients' feelings about breast surgery. *Journal of Advanced Nursing*, 18, 1710–1718.

Dane F.C. (1990) *Research Methods*. Brooks/Cole, Pacific Grove, California.

Edwards A. & Talbot R. (1994) *The Hard-Pressed Researcher*. Longman, London.

Erlandson D.A., Harris E.L., Skipper B.L. & Allen S.D. (1993) *Doing Naturalistic Inquiry*. Sage, Newbury Park, California.

Field D. (1984) We didn't want him to die on his own: nurses' accounts of nursing dying patients. *Journal of Advanced Nursing*, 9(1), 59–70.

Glaser B.G. & Strauss A.L. (1967) *The Discovery of Grounded Theory*. Aldine, Chicago.

Holloway I. (1992) Dual identities: the social reality of catering teaching. Unpublished PhD thesis, King's College, London University, London.

Kramer M. (1974) *Reality Shock: Why Nurses leave Nursing*. CV Mosby, St Louis.

Lawler J. (1991) *Behind the Screens: Nursing, Somology and the Problem of the Body*. Churchill Livingstone, Melbourne.

Lincoln Y. & Guba E. (1985) *Naturalistic Inquiry*. Sage, Beverly Hills, California.

Minichiello V., Aroni R., Timewell E. & Alexander L. (1990) *In-Depth Interviewing: Researching People*. Longman Cheshire, Melbourne.

Morse J.M. & Johnson J.L. (1991) *The Illness Experience*. Sage, Newbury Park, California.

Sandelowski M. (1994) The use of quotes in qualitative research. *Research in Nursing and Health*, **17**(6), 479–483.

Smith P. (1992) *The Emotional Labour of Nursing*. Macmillan, Basingstoke.

Strauss A. & Corbin J. (1990) *Basics of Qualitative Research: Grounded Theory Procedures and Techniques*. Sage, Newbury Park, California.

Webb C. (1992) The use of the first person in academic writing: objectivity, language and gatekeeping. *Journal of Advanced Nursing*, **17**, 747–752.

Wheeler S.J. (1989) Health visitors' and social workers' perceptions of child abuse. Unpublished BSc project, Bournemouth University, Bournemouth.

Wheeler S.J. (1992) Perceptions of child abuse. *Health Visitor* **65**(9), 316–319.

Wolcott H.F. (1990) *Writing Up Qualitative Research*. Sage, Newbury Park, California.

Wolcott H.F. (1994) *Transforming Qualitative Data: Description, Analysis, and Interpretation*. Sage, Thousand Oaks, California.

The following methodological and practical issues in qualitative research are debated here:

- Method slurring and mixing methods
- Are qualitative methods scientific?
- The importance of context
- Making inferences

Method slurring revisited

As stated before, qualitative research includes a variety of diverse approaches for the collection or analysis of data, based on different philosophical positions and rooted in various disciplines. Some are in fact philosophies rather than methods of analysis (for instance phenomenology), others present approaches to data collection, analysis and theorising such as grounded theory and ethnography. Yet others are textual analyses like discourse and conversation analysis. Even within a single method different schools compete with each other and their followers sometimes take a strong position; for instance, in grounded theory a Glaserian and a Straussian school exist (Stern, 1994; Robrecht, 1995) and in ethnography too, a variety of different approaches are used by ethnographers.

Students cannot always differentiate between methods, and some expert researchers strongly argue against 'muddling' them (Boyle *et al.*, 1991; Baker *et al.*, 1992). These writers point out that each approach in qualitative research has its own assumptions and procedures. Morse (1994) stresses that, among other factors, application and use differentiate methods and give each approach its unique character. A researcher using one of the methods should make sure that language, philosophy and strategies should 'fit' the chosen approach. Commonalities do exist, of course. Most of these approaches focus on the experiences of human beings and the perspectives of the participants, interpreted by the researcher. They uncover meanings which people give to their experiences and generally use small samples. These types of research result ultimately in a coherent story with a strong story line.

Researchers are not merely interested in the origins of these approaches (mentioned in each relevant chapter), but also in their purpose and strategies.

Grounded theory has as its aim the generation and development of theoretical ideas and focuses particularly on shared meanings in interaction. Data collection and analysis interact, and theoretical sampling takes place until saturation occurs. Through constant comparison researchers uncover the social reality of participants. In the development of grounded theory, the importance is placed on theorising specifically.

Ethnographers, on the other hand, aim to study and write about cultures. The first step for researchers is to become familiar with the setting they study and wish to research. The sample consists of key informants who possess special knowledge of these cultures. Through finding patterns and themes, the rules and rituals of cultural members are uncovered.

Phenomenologists in their turn explore the *lived experience* of participants, starting with their own reflections. The sample is selected on the basis of the people's experiences. Through the data, meanings are found which demonstrate the characteristics of a phenomenon, and meaning units are translated into statements, eventually forming the description of the phenomenon under study. Thus phenomenology gives authentic descriptions of experiences and phenomena. There are similarities here to the research process inherent in the symbolic interactionist perspective and grounded theory that we have previously described. However, as Outhwaite (1987) points out, there is a difference in focus in the approaches. Approaches within the symbolic interactionist perspective focus on interaction, and phenomenological researchers look at cognitive phenomena.

Boyle (1994) argues, that much so-called qualitative research is 'latent' or 'inferred' content analysis (Field & Morse, 1985; Wilson, 1989), but this type is criticised for not being truly qualitative. One can see that diverse pathways of qualitative research with different language use have been developed, although they cannot always be wholly separated from each other and have similar basic ideas and procedures.

One of the reasons why researchers are accused of method slurring is the way in which different writers describe a single approach but do not actually develop clearly or in detail the procedures to be adopted, or even describe the strategies they used. In fact, even one of the few 'cook books' (Riley, 1990) does not differentiate between the various styles of qualitative enquiry.

There is no doubt that qualitative researchers should know about these approaches, regardless of the method which they eventually adopt. Although methods originate in different disciplines and tend to lack a single set of theories which underlie them (Atkinson, 1995), this does not necessarily mean the use of completely different procedures. Atkinson warns about 'prescriptive treatment' of the qualitative research process and 'tightly bounded typologies'. He does not believe in their exclusivity and claims that all qualitative methods do not belong to a single paradigm.

We, too, believe that modification of data collection and analysis type is not only possible but can occasionally even be desirable. This means breaking the rules and guidelines of specific approaches. Indeed, it cannot be forgotten that methodological processes and strategies evolve over time. Sandelowski (1994) points out that rigid rules might limit the imagination and creativity. She advises, however, against 'methodological anarchy'.

Novices, however, have to learn the rules and follow the guidelines and procedures properly and in great detail, while those who become well versed and expert in a method can modify or sometimes even change these rules.

Is it science?

The question whether a particular research type is scientific or not, can be problematic as the answer cannot be given in an unambiguous, simplistic way. It is sometimes claimed that qualitative enquiry can be journalistic and gives only a superficial picture of the world under study. Qualitative researchers refute this by stressing the depth of the research and the length of the observation and interviews. This cannot be described as merely impressionistic. Hitchcock & Hughes (1989:36) maintain that qualitative research meets the criteria of science as it is 'systematic, rigorous and analytical'. Others feel differently. Clarke (1995), for example, comes to the conclusion that human relationships might be demeaned by involving scientific equations. Description of the social world cannot be truly 'scientific'. To be effective and bring about change, this type of research should be creative.

Most social science researchers agree that qualitative writing has some characteristics in common with novel writing and the arts but believe that it is scientific. Minichiello *et al.* (1990) argue that consistent and rational research cannot be labelled unscientific because it is based on a different world view from traditional forms of scientific enquiry. Systematic procedures, theorising and critical evaluation, all elements of scientific work, are involved in good qualitative research, while this is not necessarily true for the stories of journalists.

We would assert that the collection and even the interpretation of data should be rational and systematic and not arbitrary. The aim of all research, after all, is *trustworthy knowledge* (a term used by Sartori, 1994). Qualitative research should aim for this. It is difficult to adopt a stance in which science is strictly differentiated from non-science; research reflects the real world which cannot always be grasped through science alone.

The objectivity/subjectivity debate

To achieve objectivity is one of the aims in traditional, quantitative research; it is seen as one of the signs of rigour. This notion of objectivity means that the researchers try to take a neutral stance and do not let their own values impinge on the enquiry. Lindlof (1995:25) states 'scientific objectivity basically means refusing to let value positions affect the way a study is designed or the way empirical data are collected or evaluated'. Researchers distance themselves from respondents in order to avoid contaminating the data. They assume that they achieve the aim of scientific enquiry by gaining objective knowledge, free from biases. This view of science takes the world as consisting of measurable facts little affected by human beings.

We claim that the search for objectivity is not as simple as it seems. It is problematic in quantitative research but has even more complexity in qualitative enquiry. Objectivity in quantitative research emerges, so researchers claim, as a result of standardisation and distance from the participants. Streubert & Carpenter (1995) argue that the search for objectivity has some value when the phenomena studied are not human and when prediction and control are the ultimate aims of the research. Even this type of research cannot achieve complete objectivity and value neutrality: facts as seen by people are imbued with meaning; indeed the researchers bring their own values and ideas to the investigation. Choice of topic area, the type of sampling and the interpretation of data are affected by the researchers' perspectives and therefore contain elements of subjectivity.

Within nursing and health research, a number of methods are used, as mentioned before, and these cover a continuum between relatively objective and subjective perspectives. Nurses do experiments, for instance, in which subjects or subject matter are randomly assigned to particular treatments or conditions, or surveys using questionnaires or standardised interviews. The former are tightly controlled and often take place under laboratory conditions. They are generally seen as most objective because the researcher's values and background interfere least. Objectivity remains the ideal here. Munhall & Oiler Boyd (1993) claim that the term objectivity as used in quantitative research means the existence of a reality independent of the researcher. In this type of research, biases must be excluded to obtain the truth. For these reasons the voice of the researcher (the first person, 'I') is often, though not always, excluded. The research report or study is generally written in the passive form or third person.

Much nursing enquiry, like other social research, deals with human beings, and this makes achieving objectivity even more difficult. Qualitative research, particularly that which relies on in-depth interviewing, can be seen as more subjective. Thompson (1995) claims that health, in any case, has a 'strong subjective dimension'. Instead of searching for explanation, prediction and control, the qualitative researcher seeks understanding of human thought and behaviour and its interpretation. This type of nursing enquiry cannot be completely objective and neutral. The prolonged immersion of the researcher in the setting and the close relationship to the participants make value neutrality and objectivity difficult. Because it is impossible to remove subjectivity, the voice of the researcher, the first person 'I', is used when discussing one's own actions and the decision trail.

The researcher in qualitative research is the main research tool. The identities of researchers impinge on their work as they record what they hear, feel and see. They interpret the words and behaviours of the participants and do not merely recount them. LeCompte (1987) mentions bias in the biography of researchers whose membership in a group or culture affects the research process; personal beliefs and conditions also influence it. This may, of course, create biases and subjectivity but can be useful and sensitise researchers to the events and the people under investigation. Some feel that 'bias' is a misnomer because the term sounds negative, while the subjective thoughts can be a resource for the study, as long as the researchers are reflexive and aware of their own assumptions (Olesen, 1994).

Students should be warned, however, that they might not always recognise their subjectivity. Qualitative research may generate strong feelings, especially when a researcher bases a study on his or her own experience, and this can create undue bias.

> ## Example
>
> One of our students had experienced a relative's death in hospital. She felt she had been prevented from supporting her relative by officious health professionals. As an experienced nurse she was angry with colleagues and in her anger she decided to study nurses' perceptions of the role of dying patients' relatives. It took her quite a while to discuss the topic with her supervisors and to deal with her anger. She did not change her topic area because, as an experienced professional, she recognised the importance of the problem, but she managed her anger by being reflexive about it so that it did not skew the study (undergraduate experience).

Individuals cannot help bringing their own cultural and personal background to the setting; their gender, too, might influence them. Of course, they must try to be aware of their own feelings and biases and take account of their position, although it is difficult to be always conscious of one's own 'cultural baggage'. Researchers bring to the enquiry their own personalities, values and life experience and have to recognise and openly acknowledge their subjectivity.

The qualitative researcher recognises that reality is socially constructed and depends on culture, time and place as well as on the individuals who observe the situation and interpret it. 'Objective reality is grounded in our subjective experience in the world' (Munhall & Oiler Boyd, 1993: xix), so in qualitative research the subjective perspectives of participants and researcher become part of the study. The thoughts and values of the informants impinge on the research, but these are, of course, exactly that which the researchers want to explore. The investigator's own subjectivity becomes an analytic tool and is built into the research; indeed, personal reaction to the situation can become a source of data (Lipson, 1984, 1991) and subjectivity a resource. Using the self as a tool can help the researcher empathise and build relationships with the informants.

On the other hand, health professionals' own assumptions could interfere with the study. They feel they know the psychological problems that patients with certain conditions experience. A closed mind might prevent them from looking further and focusing on patients' real concerns.

Phenomenologists use *bracketing* (the term derived from Husserl, see Chapter 8), a process which they think improves the rigour of the research. This means that the researchers explore their own assumptions and preconceptions in order to set them aside rather than concealing them. Researchers must be conscious of their own subjectivity and not see it as a limitation or constraint. One of the ways to do this is the use of field notes, when biases become identified, as all experiences, feelings and thoughts are written down and become objects of reflection. The researcher must be self-critical and explicit.

'We arrive the closest we can get to an objective account of the phenomenon in question through an explanation of the ways in which the subjectivity of the researcher has structured the way it is defined in the first place.'

(Banister *et al.*, 1994:13)

The description of the methodological decisions made (the decision trail has been discussed in Chapter 12) means that readers and reviewers, as well as other researchers, can discover the subjective ideas of the investigator. That is, the research is not wholly subjective but is open to critical enquiry (Thompson, 1995: 50). Any distortions in the research because of interviewer or observer bias can thus be eliminated to some extent although total exclusion is never possible.

In some ways, the qualitative approach might even be seen as less subjective than quantitative research, because researchers do not impose a prior framework; if they are aware of their own biases and make them explicit, the readers can judge for themselves the quality of the research. This debate on objectivity and subjectivity can help us realise that there is no such thing as a single reality or truth but that multiple realities exist. Kvale (1995) writes that the concern of social scientists with objectivity may well reflect the doubts that they have about objective reality and act as an assurance that it actually exists.

Generalisability and replicability

Quantitative researchers point out that the small samples prevent the research from being generalisable. Qualitative researchers generally do not claim generalisability as they realise that they produce only a slice of the social situation rather than the whole. Generalisability can only be discussed in terms of theoretical propositions (Bryman, 1988). However, some generalisations can be made if they are supported by evidence from a number of other sources.

Morse (1994) also speaks of theory-based generalisations. She claims that theory contributes to the 'greater body of knowledge' when it is 'recontextualised' into a variety of settings. Researchers generalise because they have gained knowledge of many concepts and instances about the phenomenon that is being studied. Payne & Cuff (1982) argue that generalisations from a few cases are possible: just as a small group of statements can establish generalisations about an entire language, so individual cases can do the same for a subculture.

Qualitative research does have specificity; some writers even claim that large sample size, far from being useful, prevents examination of meaning and context (Banister *et al.*, 1994). Of course, the type of sample and sample size have to be justified. Eastabrooks *et al.* (1994) believe that, in any case, there is a way to counter criticism of qualitative research studies with relatively small homogeneous samples. These writers stress the importance of an approach that takes into account a number of these studies focusing on similar topic, populations and methods, by which generalisation, or at least typicality, can be achieved.

Qualitative researchers often, if not always, produce a description and analysis of reality that is typical for a particular setting by taking into account the conditions and the context under which the phenomena occur. Typicality is achieved when experiences and perceptions of a specific sample are typical of the phenomena under study and relate to the theoretical ideas which have emerged.

Critics of qualitative research maintain that it cannot be fully replicated by other researchers in the same way as quantitative research. This is true to the extent that the relationship between the researcher and the participant in the research is unique and can never be replicated, although the same procedures and techniques may be followed and adopted.

The importance of context

Generalisability and replicability of a study often mean that it is abstracted from the context. The context in one piece of research differs from any other, one of the reasons why it is difficult to generalise or replicate. Although context is an issue in all enquiry, it has major significance in qualitative research. Novice researchers do not always recognise this and discuss the phenomenon to be studied without taking into account the context. When they do remember it, they often mean by context the immediate environment and physical location of the people they study, and disregard the cultural and historical situation which is important for an under-standing of the phenomenon and the meaning which participants give to it.

Hinds *et al.* (1992) differentiate between the following four types of context. The immediate context is the space and environment in which interaction takes place with the focus on the present. The specific context is characterised by a variety of factors such as time of day, other people, changes in the environment, all in the immediate past. The general context concerns interpretations which have devel-oped over time, while the metacontext is the connection with the social structure and the construction of a shared social reality by participants, including the researcher. For instance, a pregnant woman is not only influenced by the proce-dures that are undertaken in hospital, but also by the people who care for her or visit, previous experiences, her personal belief system and the social and cultural background in which she is situated.

Researchers should understand the context in which the participants act and feel but must also take account of their own location in time, space and culture. The awareness of this as a basis for their own assumptions can help in understanding the meaning context of participants.

Inferential leaps and premature closure

As part of the process of validating the data analysis, researchers should check against 'inferential leaps'. The phrase inferential leap is our own and developed through supervising students. In our early days of research supervision it became apparent that students would too quickly infer conclusions from the data. In their haste to make sense of the data and develop a picture, students can too readily make inferential leaps. It seems that students remember concepts or frameworks previously learnt or discovered as a background to the research, and they try to fit these to the data. The researcher has to return to the data continually, checking and verifying so that inferential leaps are not made.

This is closely connected with the warning against 'premature closure' (Glaser, 1978) which is one of the problems of qualitative research. Often novice researchers decide on a theme or category at an early stage of the research process. In grounded theory in particular, the danger exists that once researchers have generated some theoretical ideas, they sit back and decide that they arrived at full explanations for the phenomenon under study. Sometimes there has been no full investigation of the data, sometimes they close their minds to new ideas. Morse (1994) claims that premature closure can lead to inadequate theory.

References

Atkinson P. (1995) Some perils of paradigms. *Qualitative Health Research*, 5(1), 117–124.

Baker C., Wuest J. & Stern P.N. (1992) Method slurring: the grounded theory/phenomenology example. *Journal of Advanced Nursing*, 17, 1355–1360.

Banister P., Bruman E., Parker I., Taylor M. & Tindall C. (1994) *Qualitative Methods in Psychology: A Research Guide*. Open University Press, Milton Keynes.

Boyle J. (1994) Styles of ethnography. In *Critical Issues in Qualitative Research Methods* (ed. J.M. Morse), pp. 159–185, Sage, Thousand Oaks, California.

Boyle J., Morse J.M., May K. & Hutchinson S. (1991) Dialogue. On muddling methods. In *Critical Issues in Qualitative Research Methods* (ed. J.M. Morse), p. 257, Sage, Thousand Oaks, California.

Bryman A. (1988) *Quantity and Quality in Social Research*. Unwin Hyman, London.

Clarke L. (1995) Nursing research: science, visions and telling stories. *Journal of Advanced Nursing*, 21, 584–593.

Field P.A. & Morse J.M. (1985) *Nursing Research: The Application of Qualitative Approaches*. Croom Helm, London.

Glaser B. G. (1978) *Theoretical Sensitivity*. Sociology Press, Mill Valley, California.

Hinds P., Chaves D.E. & Cypess S.M. (1992) Context as a source of meaning and understanding. *Qualitative Health Research*, 2(1), 61–74.

Hitchcock G. & Hughes D. (1989) *Research and the Teacher: A Qualitative Introduction to School-Based Research*. Routledge, London.

Kvale S. (1995) The social construction of validity. *Qualitative Inquiry*, 1(1), 19–40.

LeCompte M.D. (1987) Bias in the biography: bias and subjectivity in ethnographic research. *Anthropology and Education Quarterly*, 18(1), 43–52.

Lindlof T.R. (1995) *Qualitative Communication Research Methods*. Sage, Thousand Oaks, California.

Lipson J. G. (1984) Combining researcher clinical and personal roles: enrichment or confusion. *Human Organisation* 43(4), 348–352.

Lipson J.G. (1991) The use of self in ethnographic research. In *Critical Issues in Qualitative Research Methods* (ed. J.M. Morse), pp. 73–89, Sage, Thousand Oaks, California.

Minichiello V., Aroni R., Tinewall E. & Alexander L. (1990) *In-depth Interviewing: Researching People*. Longman Chesire, Melbourne.

Morse J. (1994) 'Emerging from the data': the cognitive processes of analysis in qualitative inquiry. In *Critical Issues in Qualitative Research Methods* (ed. J.M. Morse), pp. 23–43, Sage, Thousand Oaks, California.

Munhall P.L. & Oiler Boyd C. (1993) *Nursing Research: A Qualitative Perspective*. National League for Nursing Press, New York.

Olesen V. (1994) Feminism and models of qualitative research. In *Handbook of Qualitative Research*. (eds N.K. Denzin & Y.S. Lincoln), pp. 158–174, Sage, Thousand Oaks, California.

Outhwaite W. (1987) *New Philosophies of Social Science Realism: Hermeneutics and Critical Theory*. Macmillan Education, Basingstoke.

Payne G.C.F. & Cuff E.C. (1982) *Doing Teaching*. Batsford, London.

Riley J. (1990) *Getting the Most from your Data. A Handbook of Practical Ideas on How to Analyse Qualitative Data*. Technical and Educational Services Ltd, Bristol.

Robrecht L.C. (1995) Grounded theory: evolving methods. *Qualitative Health Research*, 5(2), 169–177.

Sandelowski M. (1994) The proof is in the pottery: toward a poetic for qualitative inquiry. In *Critical Issues in Qualitative Research Methods* (ed. J.M. Morse), pp. 46–63, Sage, Thousand Oaks, California.

Sartori D. (1994) Women's authority in science. In *Knowing the Difference: Feminist Perspectives in Epistemology* (eds K. Lennon & M. Whitford), pp. 110–121, Routledge, London.

Stern P.N. (1994) Eroding grounded theory. In *Critical Issues in Qualitative Research Methodology* (ed. J.M. Morse), pp. 212–223, Sage, Thousand Oaks, California.

Streubert H.J. & Carpenter D.R. (1995) *Qualitative Research in Nursing: Advancing the Humanistic Perspective*. J.B. Lippincott, Philadelphia.

Thompson N. (1995) *Theory and Practice in Health and Social Care*. Open University Press, Milton Keynes.

Wilson H.S. (1989) The craft of qualitative analysis. In *Research in Nursing* 2nd edn (ed. H.S. Wilson), pp. 394–428, Addison Wesley, Menlo Park, California.

Chapter 15

Computers in Qualitative Research

A brief summary will be given here on computer use in qualitative research with an outline of the following:

- When to use computers
- Advantages and problems
- Computer approaches to qualitative analysis
- The functions of the computer

As we are not experts in this field we shall only give an overview and references for further study.

In the past, qualitative researchers depended for their analysis to a large extent on cutting, sorting and pasting bits of paper. This meant that the researcher was left with a mass of paper cuttings, a great many boxes and envelopes and/or an elaborate card system. Computers have been used in the analysis of qualitative data mainly since the 1980s (Lee & Fielding, 1991). Some researchers believed then, that computing skills were not only unnecessary but that their use could make qualitative research mechanistic and rigid, the very characteristics which might change its lively humanistic nature.

Even now there are some who think this. For instance, Becker (1993) warns the grounded theorist about the use of computers. Becker feels that computers might prevent sensitivity to the data and the discovery of meanings. Computers might distance researchers from the data. In nursing and midwifery research where emotional engagement and sensitivity is necessary, the use of computers could be problematic.

Nevertheless, in the last 10 years, most researchers have felt that computers can be useful and make the process of qualitative research less cumbersome. Managing a large volume of data by hand is boring and tiring because the search for specific ideas, words, incidents or events takes time. Glesne & Peshkin (1992:145) call the computer 'a tool for executing the mechanical or clerical task of qualitative research'.

Depending on their own stance towards research, or their individual needs, nurses can, of course, choose whether or not to use computer programs. The type of approach influences the program for analysis of qualitative data.

Who and when?

Most students already use word processors for entering and storing data. Word processing programs create and revise text and can therefore be helpful to researchers in the transcription of interviews and field notes and in writing the report. It is essential that students learn word processing skills because correcting a text on the machine takes much less time than rewriting by hand or typewriter.

Many researchers would like to learn the use of computers for qualitative analysis, but the practicalities of this must be sorted out before starting a project. The usefulness of computers depends on the researchers' initial knowledge of computers as well as the time-span and size of the project. Some of our students started learning to use the computer for data analysis and found it impossible to do within the allocated time.

Miles & Weitzman (1994) speak of levels of computer skills. Level 1 users have limited knowledge of computers. They use a word processing program efficiently, including creating, cutting and pasting text. We would suggest that the students who have a short time to finish a project might be better advised to start the process of analysis manually, using the computer knowledge they already possess rather than learning new and complex processes. Our undergraduate students generally only have around 9 months for their project, and the time is too short for mastering a complex package; effort and energy are better expanded in listening to tapes, organising the data and thinking about them.

PhD students with several years' research work ahead would do well to learn computer skills to help in the analysis of qualitative data. There is the likelihood that it will be possible for them to apply their knowledge in future research projects. Level 1 researchers who are interested in using computers are advised to consider user friendly programs and get help from others who have some expertise.

Level 2 users can cope with a variety of programs, and they should select one which is appropriate to their research. If they are planning a long-term project, they can choose a complex package. Miles & Weitzman (1994) advise researchers to consult experienced users of qualitative data analysis packages, but some guidelines and textbooks on the use of computers in qualitative research also detail the practical processes.

Researchers at level 3 are interested and knowledgeable computer users and quickly acquire expertise in the program they need for their research. Level 4 computer users (individuals who are never far away from their machine) have expert knowledge and experience of computing and computer packages. They will have no difficulties dealing with programs for qualitative research. We would advise the use of a computer program for analysis if the nurse researcher has a large sample (for qualitative research around 40 interviewees for instance, would be a large sample) and a long time-span, because the data can be managed more efficiently.

We found it difficult to learn the use of computer packages for qualitative analysis from manuals, although some people seem to be able to do so. It is always easier to let expert users teach us rather than relying on a manual, but one must be aware that very experienced users might be too far advanced to use beginners' terms and explain the skills in a simple way. They take the language and skills needed for computers for granted. It is far better to have a teacher who is just a few steps ahead.

Russell & Gregory (1993) point out that researchers perform both mechanical and conceptual roles in the analysis of data. Not only do researchers store and retrieve data, which are mechanical activities, but they also group, code and categorise, tasks which involve conceptual activity. These two types of activities are always linked to each other and can both be helped by the use of computers.

Advantages and problems

Researchers use computers as tools for facilitating processes that were done manually in the past, but it is a fallacy to believe that data can be analysed more quickly by computer programs, because it takes time to learn their use. Once learnt though, they can save time and help researchers to be more organised and systematic and facilitate planning. Data are more accessible and fewer hours are spent sorting and coding the data. Cutting and pasting is easy, and more time can be given to thinking through the analysis. Students should remember to back up their data by storing copies on floppy discs or other computers.

Tesch (1993) states that the introduction of computers in qualitative research does not mean a complete change in the process of analysis, but the new tool can make it easier and more flexible. While decisions and judgments are still made by the researcher, searching, cutting and pasting is done by machine. Computers cannot formulate categories or interpret the data, but they can make the analysis more accurate and comprehensive.

Certain problems emerge, however, when using computers. Seidel (1991:107), one of the major proponents of computer use in qualitative analysis, warns of 'analytic madness'; he states that the use of technology may be a problem which can interfere with appropriate qualitative analysis. He lists three major issues. First, when researchers' ideas have their roots in the quantitative perspective, they are tempted to collect and manage more data than necessary. The overload of data might prevent researchers from looking for the most interesting and significant ideas. Instead of searching for deeper meaning in the data, they try to make up for the lack of depth by focusing on the volume of data.

The second issue concerns the relationship between researchers and data. This might become mechanistic if analysts do not see the need to examine and evaluate the data carefully. The number of instances of a code or category is often seen as more important than a single significant occurrence just because counting is easy. The lack of scrutiny might prevent the researcher from seeing the real meaning of the phenomenon under study. This sometimes happens when the data are analysed manually but the danger becomes greater through the use of computers.

The distancing of the researcher from the data is another problem in the use of computers. The involvement with a file on a computer or a printed sheet of paper which is coded by machine seems less personal than coding and categorising by hand. In spite of these potential problems many well-known qualitative researchers use computer programs when conducting a major piece of research. Seidel himself is the inventor and developer of the much-used computer package *Ethnograph* which helps researchers to identify and retrieve text from documents.

Approaches to qualitative analysis

Tesch (1993) describes three main approaches to qualitative data analysis but acknowledges that these groupings and their subgroups are not neat and discrete, they overlap and do not reflect reality. Both the content of the text and the process of communication are seen as important.

Language-oriented types of analysis are used by researchers who are primarily interested in language and its meaning, examples are conversation and discourse analysis as well as ethnography. These approaches focus not only on words and verbal interaction but also on the way in which people make sense of their world.

Descriptive/interpretive approaches deal with narratives and give descriptions of feelings and actions. Examples are life histories and certain types of ethnographies which are descriptions and interpretations of a culture. Researchers tell stories and provide interpretations of meanings which participants in the research attach to their experiences.

In theory-building, the researcher finds patterns and links between ideas and attempts to build theory. From insights generated by the data, general principles often emerge. This is more explanatory than other approaches. Grounded theory represents this type of research. Richards & Richards (1994) stress that the process of theory building is not mechanical but demands creativity from the researcher.

The tasks of the computer

Tesch (1993) lists a variety of tasks, formerly done manually, which can now be performed by computers:

Storing and retrieving texts

Storing and retrieving texts such as interview transcripts, field notes or diaries is the most common use of computer programs in qualitative research. Data are easily accessible, for instance interview transcripts and field notes can be stored in separate files and memos attached to the category to which they belong, and called upon when needed. Researchers must always label and date these files to keep order among them. Warning: Copies of files should be made on floppy discs and stored safely in a different location.

Locating words, phrases or segments of data in the text

Researchers might want to find particular words or phrases and the context in which they occur as well as their frequency. Sentences and paragraphs as well as specific key words can be recalled. These can indicate the importance which informants and researcher attach to particular words or concepts (though it is dangerous to rely on the number of instances rather than an in-depth examination of each instance).

Naming or labelling sections of data

These labels are key words which define an idea, or they can be summaries of the content of the data. Categorising starts here and is based on this labelling. Categories are concepts attached to a topic emerging from the data and a step in their interpretation. Researchers give the appropriate label to each segment of data or to instances that belong together. Revision of names in the light of further analysis then becomes less difficult. The creation of categories from the data is a step towards theory building.

Sorting and organising data segments

This is sorting and organising the data segments and topic units according to the named categories or key words attached to them. Organising data into segments (bits, chunks or strips as they are sometimes called) means dividing them into discrete units (although these can sometimes overlap with each other). All segments with the same inherent themes or categories can be grouped together.

Identifying data units

This means identifying data units relevant to several categories and discovering relationships between them. Researchers always try to see a structure and links between categories. These links can be found more easily in and across particular files. This helps in the development of working hypotheses, models or typologies. Of course, none of these processes are done by the computer, they are based on the researcher's theoretical considerations and decision making but helped by the machine. Each proposition can be checked out. For instance, a nurse researcher may discover from examining the data that elderly patients are compliant with district nurses' advice. This can be checked quickly through viewing the categories and the links between them.

Preparing diagrams

Diagrams illustrate the relationship between themes or categories. The graphic display can enhance the story line and help to convey its meaning. Many of our students clarify their findings by showing links and connections through diagrams.

Extracting quotes

Quotes can be extracted from the informants' words or field notes for insertion in the final story. Most qualitative researchers use quotes when they write up their study. These are excerpts from the data to give evidence that their discussion has its basis in the data themselves. The quotes enhance the story line, that is, they make the story more lively and interesting.

Since the early 1980s, when the journal *Qualitative Sociology* (1984, 7, 1–2) published a special edition on the use of computers in qualitative research, new ideas and packages have been developed. Some programs are more sophisticated than others. Each has its own technical traits depending on the choice of the designer. For students who wish to use this software, it is essential to become familiar with it.

For further information and details on particular programmes, we advise researchers to look at the text books by Fielding & Lee (1991), Tesch (1993), Weitzman & Miles (1994) and Dey (1993). In these, programs and addresses can be found. The two best known British texts are those of Fielding & Lee and Dey.

Computers in qualitative research have largely been accepted. In fact some funding agencies are impressed by computer packages because they are used to computers in survey research. The greatest help from computers lies in the management of data, because 'good analysis requires efficient management of one's data' (Dey, 1993:74).

Summary

Computers are now used more often in qualitative research than in the past. They are useful in cutting down the mechanical procedures while decisions are still made by the researcher. A number of computer packages exist for different purposes and different makes of computer. In general, computers are used for storing and retrieving texts and locating segments as well as naming and sorting the data. Data units can be identified more easily. This shows that the tasks of computers consist, in the main, of the efficient management of the data.

References

Becker P.H. (1993) Common pitfalls in grounded theory research. *Qualitative Health Research*, 3(2), 254–260.

Dey I. (1993) *Qualitative Data Analysis*. Routledge, London.

Fielding N.G. & Lee R.M. (1991) *Using Computers in Qualitative Research*. Sage, London.

Glesne C. & Peshkin A. (1992) *Becoming Qualitative Researchers: An Introduction*. Longman, New York.

Lee R.M. & Fielding N.G. (1991) Computing for qualitative research: options, problems and potential. In *Using Computers in Qualitative Research* (eds N. Fielding & R.M. Lee), pp. 1–13, Sage, London.

Miles M.B. & Weitzman E.A. (1994) Choosing computer programs for qualitative data analysis. In *Qualitative Data Analysis* 2nd edn, (eds M.B. Miles & A.M. Huberman), pp. 311–330, Sage, Thousand Oaks, California.

Richards T.J. & Richards L. (1994) Using computers in qualitative research. In *Handbook of Qualitative Research* (eds N. Denzin & Y. Lincoln), pp. 445–462, Sage, Thousand Oaks, California.

Russell C.K. & Gregory D.M. (1993) Issues for consideration when choosing a qualitative data management system. *Journal of Advanced Nursing*, **18**, 1806–1816.

Seidel J. (1991) Method and madness in the application of computer technology to qualitative data analysis. In *Using Computers in Qualitative Research* (eds N.G. Fielding & R.M. Lee), pp. 107–118, Sage, London.

Tesch R. (1993) Personal computers in qualitative research. In *Ethnography and Qualitative Design in Educational Research* 2nd edn, pp. 279–314, Academic Press, Chicago.

Weitzman E.A. & Miles M.B. (1994) *Computer Aided Qualitative Data Analysis: A Review of Selected Software.* Center for Policy Research, New York.

Chapter 16

Supervision of Qualitative Research

We shall address the following issues in this chapter which is intended for students:

- Single or joint supervision?
- The tasks of students and supervisors
- The practical aspects of supervision

Student projects need to be supervised, and students are often concerned about the problem of choice concerning supervisors and the relationship they develop with each other. Although supervision may differ according to circumstances, that is, the type of research and the topic as well as the level of study and experience of students, the principles remain similar for different students and types of research.

Howard & Sharp (1983) claim that supervisors have some responsibility for the standard and completion of the research and for ensuring that students define and achieve aims and objectives. Supervisors have an obligation to the student to support and advise. However, the ultimate responsibility lies with the students, and they are in charge of their own research.

Sometimes students can choose their own supervisors, after deciding on the research topic, from a given list of potential tutors which contains their specific interests. The freedom to choose is important for both student and supervisor since each needs to feel comfortable with the topic and the relationship. Sometimes a programme leader allocates supervisors according to their particular expertise. They are selected on the basis of their knowledge of research methods and/or because of their knowledge of the topic.

Sometimes students choose a tutor with whom they can work, who is seen as helpful and supportive or whom they respect as a knowledgeable professional. Perhaps this is the most useful criterion, as the students will eventually become expert in their own research. For supervisors, too, the selection process is important because of the close connections that they will develop over time.

There is a need to match the style of supervisors and students. Some students, for example, like having a highly structured timetable and want to be directed or organised by their supervisors, others are self-directed and see supervisors as an informal sounding board.

Single or joint supervision?

Students have either one or two supervisors for their research studies. One supervisor could be an expert in the research method, the other might have specialist knowledge in the field of study; supervisors generally differ in their skills and knowledge but complement each other.

There are a number of arguments for joint supervision; it safeguards both student and tutor. For the student, continuity is ensured when one supervisor is absent or ill. The student experience can be enhanced by the support of two supervisors. For the supervisors there is support from colleagues who can discuss the appropriateness of advice about which they are uncertain. New supervisors gain from the guidance of experienced colleagues.

The case for single supervision is not as strong. The main argument relates to the clear guidance of students who do not receive conflicting guidance from different people if there is just one adviser. In universities and colleges where staff move frequently, students will be safer with two supervisors. To avoid conflicting advice to students, it is, of course, important that joint supervisors have a common ideology about supervision, a similar view about the particular method and topic, and that they stay in contact with each other. Students must be aware of some of the pitfalls and problems in supervision, because ultimately the responsibility is theirs.

It is important to choose supervisors who do not denigrate one type of method at the expense of another, although students will grasp that the division between qualitative and quantitative methods is based on different ways of thinking and different paradigms; as Allan (1991:177) states: 'the contrast runs deeper than data-processing procedures'. Students often propose an ambitious project in which they intend to use both qualitative and quantitative methods, while it might be better to follow Leininger's (1992) advice and triangulate within a method, for instance through the use of both qualitative (unstructured or semi-structured) interviews and participant observation. For short student projects which take less than a year, between-method triangulation is too time consuming although occasionally a student will successfully complete a project using between-method triangulation.

Supervisors have the task of asking questions about the particular circumstances, settings and people which the students want to take into account when investigating the topic. Often they have knowledge of specific methodologies and are able to advise students on relevant and useful method texts. Although students cannot be forced to listen to their supervisors, they will usually find it profitable to do so.

Kane (1985) claims that researchers have a duty to their discipline and should report data truthfully, accurately and as completely as possible. The ethical rules of fidelity and veracity are very important in establishing a trusting relationship. In this process truth telling is essential. There is an obvious duty for both researcher and supervisor to recognise the need to share all aspects of the study phases, be they positive or negative.

Supervisors are able to help because they have inside knowledge of the research and often spot distortions. In general supervisors have lengthy experience of a variety of student projects. This knowledge helps students to trust the advice given and be guided appropriately.

The tasks of students and supervisors

Supervisors and students have a common aim, that is to achieve a study of high standard which will be completed on time. Both student and supervisor(s) should be committed to the contract of respectively doing and supporting the research. The supervisor generally guides and advises rather than directs, except in circumstances where the student acts contrary to ethical and research guidelines.

The ground rules are negotiated by supervisor and student at the very beginning of the relationship. The frequency of contact depends on the student's needs and the stage in the research process. This can be negotiated at the beginning of the research and revised at intervals. Generally the student needs most help and support at the start and then again at the stage of writing up. Nevertheless, it is necessary for students to be in touch regularly rather than in irregular and erratic contact. Some people need to see the supervisor often, others enjoy working on their own, though they too need feedback and constructive criticism. There should be a systematic and structured programme of work which forms the basis for the student–supervisor work relationship, but the instigation for this programme should come from students themselves.

The responsibility for contacting supervisors rests largely with students. Telephone contact can be useful, especially when a student experiences an academic or even a personal problem which affects the smooth process of the research.

Howard & Sharp (1983) advise that students inform the supervisor in advance of a meeting about the questions and problems they have. This means that both students and supervisor are prepared for the meeting which saves precious time for the participants. Many students and supervisors keep written notes on the supervision meetings; this is useful as a basis for further appointments and makes meetings more systematic and methodical. The supervisor generally advises the student to come with questions and problems. Most supervisors become involved and interested in the students' research topics. Students have the right to expect this interest.

Students do not always want to start writing after the start of the data collection; they believe that much of the research is 'in their head'. In our experience this is a fallacy, and it is useful to start writing early. The supervisor often asks for chapters on background, literature review and methodology, depending on the type of research. This ensures that students not only understand the process but also produce some ideas which generate fresh motivation and interest, even though sections of the writing might have to be changed at a later stage. This way students immerse themselves in the methodology, and some of the problems and pitfalls of the research become obvious and can be resolved at an early stage.

Often students are so enthusiastic about the research that they start data collection and analysis before being acquainted with the research methods. This can lead to inadequate interviewing and observation because guidelines for the method have been neglected. Students must make sure that they are fully aware of the strategies, techniques and problems of their chosen research method. Indeed, students sometimes need a break so they can reflect on methods and topic.

Students sometimes find that the writing up at the end is an insurmountable task. The advice to start writing early will lessen this problem. The introduction, research strategies and writing up of ethical considerations, might give direction to later chapters, and can be written quite early. If written work is sent to supervisors before a meeting, they are then able to give feedback and encouragement more easily. Students can expect that their supervisors have read the written work when they come for their pre-arranged supervision sessions, and that it will be criticised constructively. Sometimes supervisors may send their comments in writing to students before the meeting.

Phillips & Pugh (1987) suggest that the script becomes the basis for discussion. It is inadvisable to leave writing to the last stage of the research for two reasons: interesting and stimulating ideas will be forgotten, and students might run out of time and hence panic. Seeing a chunk of the report in writing will motivate the student to proceed. All through, researchers make field notes and memos as often as possible. The usefulness of carrying a small writing pad, to jot down ideas when they arise unexpectedly, cannot be underestimated.

Supervisors are not always gentle and diplomatic in their criticism; some students are easily hurt by it, but the advice is best taken without seeing it as a personal attack but as an academic argument. In any case the relationship between supervisor and student develops over time as they learn about each others' weaknesses, strengths and idiosyncrasies, and both sides negotiate the process. The supervisors who are best able to provide a structure for students, draw out their ideas and are flexible and approachable, thus creating an open learning climate (Phillips & Pugh, 1987), but if students lack this type of supervisor, they can still learn.

Supervisors cannot always help their students because they do not have unlimited knowledge about all the facets of the research. Students often find other experts who can advise them, and on whose knowledge they can draw without offending the supervisor. Indeed, supervisors often know their own limitations and help students find other experts.

Students build up relationships with their supervisors on a one-to-one basis. Eventually the student becomes an independent researcher and expert in the field of study and the supervisor acts as an adviser who takes a critical stance to the work.

We would argue that supervision is an essential component of research work and a very important aspect of establishing rigour and trustworthiness in the study.

Some practical considerations

There are some other practical points which must be remembered. Students should make an appointment before coming to see their supervisors if this is at all possible. Of course, open access to supervision is sometimes necessary and always valuable, but supervisors are busy and an appointment system helps to save time for all parties. Students (and supervisors) should be available and punctual for the pre-arranged meeting, but if appointments need to be cancelled, the cancellation should be made as early as possible. If no other time for necessary supervision can be found, an occasional telephone session might do in an emergency. The main stress should be on regular and quality time of contact.

Summary

Student and supervisor(s) have responsibility for the research project, but the main responsibility for the research lies with the student. Supervisors are chosen because of their knowledge in the area of methodology and topic. Negotiation between students and supervisors takes place early in the research when the ground rules are established.

It is essential that close and regular contact is maintained between the student and the supervisor(s) and that they share ideas throughout the research.

Acknowledgement

This chapter was published in an extended version in: Holloway I.M. (1995) Supervising student projects: the case of qualitative research. *Nurse Education Todoay* **15**, 257–262, published by Churchill Livingstone, Edinburgh.

References

Allan G. (1991) Qualitative research In *Handbook for Research Students in the Social Sciences* (eds G. Allan & C. Skinner), pp. 177–189, Falmer Press, London.

Howard K. & Sharp J.A. (1983) *The Management of a Student Research Project*. Gower, Aldershott.

Kane E. (1985) *Doing Your Own Research*. Marion Boyars, London.

Leininger M. (1992) Current issues, problems, and trends to advance qualitative paradigmatic research methods for the future. *Qualitative Health Research*, 2(4), 392–415.

Phillips E.M. & Pugh D.S. (1987) *How to get a PhD*. Open University Press, Milton Keynes.

Glossary

A priori: Thinking in which propositions and assumptions precede and direct the research.

Abstract: Brief summary of the major points of the research which appears at the very beginning of the study.

Aide mémoire: Key words or questions which remind the researcher of areas of interest for the research in an in-depth interview.

Analytic induction: A procedure which makes inferences from the specific to find general rules or theories.

Appendix (appendices (pl.)): Additional material at the end of the study. It is not included in the word limit and features after the bibliography.

Assumption: Belief which has not been scientifically verified.

Auditability: Research is auditable if readers or other researchers can follow the methodological processes of the first researcher.

Audit trail (or decision trail): A detailed explanation of the thought and action processes of the researcher to help the reader understand the logic and development of the research path.

Authenticity: A term which is used to demonstrate that the findings of a research project are true.

Bias: A distortion or error in the data collection or analysis which has its origin in strongly held values or in the very presence of an observer or interviewer.

Bracketing: Holding assumptions and presuppositions in suspension.

Category: A group of concepts and ideas which have similar characteristics.

Coding (analysing): Examining and breaking down the data. Assigning a name (or a number) to a specific datum.

Concept: An abstract or generalised idea.

Constant comparison (in grounded theory): Qualitative data analysis where each datum is compared with every other piece of the data.

Construct: A construct encompasses a number of concepts or categories. The term is often used for a major category which has evolved from the reduction of a number of smaller categories.

Core category (in grounded theory): A concept which links with all other categories in the project and integrates the data.

Criterion (criteria (pl.)): A standard by which something is evaluated.

Decision trail: See audit trail.

Deduction: Proceeding from a general principle or assumption which is tested and used to explain specific phenomena or cases.

Emic perspective: The insider's point of view about their own experiences.

Epistemology: The theory of knowledge, concerned with the ways in which we know the world.

Ethnography: Research which is concerned with a description of a culture or group and the members' experiences and interpretations.

Etic perspective: The outsider's view, the perspective of the researcher.

Exhaustive description: Writing which aims to capture and describe the intensity and depth of the participants' experiences.

Field notes: A record of the observations of researchers 'in the field' while collecting data through interviews or observation.

Fieldwork: Fieldwork is the collection of data outside the laboratory.

Focus group: A group of people with similar experiences from whom researchers collect data simultaneously through interviews which are focused on the research question.

Focused interview: The interview questions become progressively more focused on emerging and relevant issues. The first interview is unstructured and broad but later interviews become more narrow and specific.

Funnelling: The process of interviewing starts with a broad basis and becomes progressively more specific during the interview process (see focused interview).

Gatekeepers: Those individuals that have the power to permit access to an organisation, a setting or people in the setting.

Generalisability: The extent to which the findings of the study can be applied to other events, settings or groups in the population.

Grounded theory: A research method which uses inductive and deductive approaches to generate theory from the data through constant comparison.

Heterogeneity: The extent to which units of a sample are dissimilar.

Homogeneity: The extent to which units of a sample are similar.

Hypothesis: An assumption which can be tested, verified and falsified.

Idiographic methods: The study of individual, unique persons or events. Research in which the individual case has primacy.

Induction: A reasoning process in which researchers proceed from the specific and concrete statements to general and abstract principles.

Informant (in qualitative research): A person who is a member of the group under study, participates in the research and helps the researcher to interpret the culture of the group.

Interview guide: Loosely formed questions which are used flexibly by the interviewer in qualitative in-depth interviews.

Interview schedule: Standardised questions which are used by a quantitative researcher in the same sequence and wording for each respondent.

Latent content analysis: A type of analysis which identifies major themes in an interview or text.

Member check: The data and interpretations are checked and verified by the informants themselves.

Method: Strategies and techniques for collecting data.

Methodology: The theories and principles on which particular methods are based.

Narrative: The description of an experience. Generally the reconstruction of informants' lives or illness experiences.

Nomothetic methods: The search for lawlike generalities or rule-following behaviour which subsume individual cases.

Objectivity: A neutral and unbiased stance.

Ontology: A branch of philosophy concerned with the nature of being.

Paradigm: A theoretical perspective or approach which is recognised by a community of scientists (including social scientists).

Phenomenology: A research approach which explores the meaning of individuals' lived experiences through their description.

Pilot study: A small-scale trial run of a research interview or observation.

Positivism: A direction in the philosophy of social science which aims to find general laws and regularities based on observation and experiment parallel to the methods of the natural sciences.

Premature closure: Arriving too early at explanation or theoretical ideas.

Progressive focusing: See funnelling.

Proposition: A working hypothesis which consists of linked concepts and establishes some regularities.

Purposive (or purposeful) sampling: A sample of key people, specific individuals chosen by pre-determined criteria which are relevant to the research question.

Reliability: The ability of a research tool to achieve consistent results.

Reflexivity: Looking back over the research process. Self-examination of the researcher.

Saturation: Sampling until no new categories emerge and all the elements of all categories are accounted for.

Story line: An analytic description and overview of the story.

Subjectivity: A personal view.

Symbolic interactionism: An interpretive approach in sociology which focuses on the meaning in interaction.

Theoretical sampling (in grounded theory): Sampling which proceeds on the basis of emerging, relevant concepts and is directed by developing theory.

Theoretical sensitivity (concept developed by Glaser): Sensitivity and awareness of the researcher to detect meaning in the data.

Theory: A set of interrelated concepts and propositions which explain social phenomena.

Thick description (concept developed by Geertz): Dense and detailed description which gives a picture of events and actions within the social context.

Triangulation: The combination of different data collection strategies, methods of research, interviewers or theoretical perspectives in the study of one phenomenon (e.g. qualitative and quantitative methods, interviews and observation).

Validity: The extent to which the researcher's findings are accurate, reflect the purpose of the study and represent reality.

Verification: Empirical validation after testing a hypothesis.

Index

abstracts
  research proposals, 26
  research write up, 173–4
access issues, 30–37, 43–5, 66–7
action research, 155–6, 159
analytic philosophy, 115–16
androcentricity, 137–8
anonymity, ethics, 46–7
anthropology, 2, 82, 83
audit, *see* evaluation criteria
audit (decision) trail, 163, 167, 168, 171–2
autonomy principle, 39, 43, 68

bias in research, *see* objectivity/subjectivity
    debate
body movement, conversation analysis,
    153–5
bracketing, phenomenology, 118, 190
BSP (basic social-psychological process),
    106

Cartesian dualism, 117
case study research, 156–8
chain referral sampling, 76, 167
Colaizzi method, phenomenological
    research, 124–8, 165–6
computers, 110, 195–200
confidentiality, ethics, 46
confirmability, 163, 168
consciousness-raising, 138–9
consent forms, 36, 44
  see also informed consent
consequential ethical theory, 40–41
context, importance of, 192
continental philosophy, 115, 116
  see also phenomenology
convenience sampling, 77
conventional ethnography, 83
conversation analysis, 153–5
counselling, role conflict, 47, 48
credibility, 163, 164–6, 167, 168
criterion-based sampling, 74

  see also purposeful sampling
critical ethnography, 83
culture, ethnographic study, 82–4

data, primacy of, 6
data analysis
  collection and, 9, 102
  computers, 110, 196–9
  ethnography, 92–3
  focus groups, 149–50, 151
  grounded theory, 101, 102–10, 111, 177,
    193
    coding and categorising, 101, 104–7
    field notes, 102, 108–9
    formal theory, 107, 108
    literature reviews, 103, 108, 111
    memos, 109–10
    substantive theory, 107–8
    theoretical sampling, 103–4, 110
    theoretical sensitivity, 102–3
  inferential leaps, 192–3
  latent content analysis, 150
  method slurring, 186–7
  phenomenology, 124–8, 165–6
  premature closure, 193
  research write up, 177, 179
data collection, 53–70
  analysis and, 9, 102
  ethnography, 84–5, 89–91
  feminist research, 139–40
  focus groups, 148
  from documents, 66–8
  grounded theory, 101–2
  interviews, 53–9, 69–70
  life histories, 61
  method slurring, 186–7
  narratives, 59–61
  observation, 61–5
  research write up, 176–7
data management
  anonymity, 46–7
  computers, 195–200